D0052920

A GOOD ENOUGH LIFE
The Dying Speak

Other books by Susan Gabori

In Search of Paradise: The Odyssey of an Italian Family

Blind Sacrifice: Portraits of Murderers

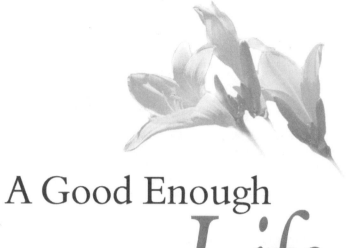

A Good Enough
Life

the dying | speak

SUSAN GABORI

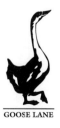

GOOSE LANE

Copyright © Susan Gabori, 2002.

All rights reserved. No part of this work may be reproduced or used in any form
or by any means, electronic or mechanical, including photocopying, recording,
or any retrieval system, without the prior written permission of the publisher.
Any requests for photocopying of any part of this book should be directed in
writing to the Canadian Copyright Licensing Agency.

Cover photo: Yellow day lilies, copyright © Roger J. Smith, 2001.
Cover and interior book design by Julie Scriver.
Printed in Canada by AGMV Marquis.
10 9 8 7 6 5 4 3 2 1

National Library of Canada Cataloguing in Publication Data

Gabori, Susan, 1947-
A good enough life : the dying speak / Susan Gabori.
Includes bibliographical references
ISBN 0-86492-352-X
1. Terminally ill — Psychology. 2. Death — Psychological aspects.
I. Title.

BF789.D4G33 2002   155.9'37   C2002-903378-0

Published with the financial support of the Canada Council for the Arts,
the Government of Canada through the Book Publishing Industry Development
Program, and the New Brunswick Culture and Sports Secretariat.

Goose Lane Editions
469 King Street
Fredericton, New Brunswick
CANADA E3B 1E5
www.gooselane.com

Look around:
look how it all leaps alive —
where death is! Alive!
He speaks truly who speaks the shade.
— Paul Celan, "Speak, You Also"
Translated by Michael Hamburger

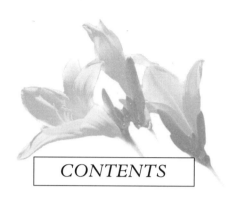

CONTENTS

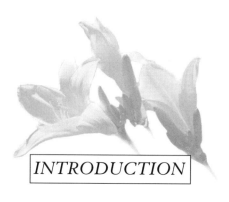

INTRODUCTION

Philosophers, psychologists, and mystics have claimed that crisis is an opportunity for growth, and certainly a diagnosis of terminal illness qualifies as a major crisis in a person's life. Bruno Bettelheim wrote in *Surviving and Other Essays* that "it is death that endows life with its deepest, most unique meaning." In that case, what can the dying teach us about living? I wanted to find people who were squeezed into a tight corner, pressed against the wall, or as the poet Paul Celan wrote, driven to the "inmost recesses" of the self. What did they find there?

In *A Good Enough Life* are portraits of twelve people who are a year to a week from death, individuals who must face themselves, confront their lives, and reflect on their imminent end. Although these are radically different lives, certain realizations and understandings echo from one portrait to another. Each story is filled with extraordinary struggles and hardships, as well as with surprising honesty and joy at what has been discovered in this last phase of life.

In these interviews, I felt like a miner going into the dark depths of the earth in search of treasure. I didn't know what I would find, but I knew that whatever was revealed would be precious. Questions evoked memories, leading to more questions. I asked about the painful events in these people's lives that triggered anger, worry, or fear. What had made them suffer? Why?

Having trained as a filmmaker and worked as a cameraman at the National Film Board in Montreal, I saw these portraits in visual terms — some areas were fully lit, others were lit for shadow, while the rest was still incomplete. Portraiture is a strong tradition in painting, drawing, and photography, and *A Good Enough Life* is portraits in words. Terminal illness is the critical point where a life's threads converge, where dramatic shifts can occur. I did not attempt to include everything but focused on meaningful moments, painful truths, crucial relationships, and key realizations. Also, the mixture of tragedy and humour in certain lives fascinated me.

As in portrait painting, there is a connection between background and subject. In the interviews, I explore the relationship between the psyche and its setting, paying attention to place, time, and colour. For this reason, the portraits in *A Good Enough Life* are also about history, memory, and psychology. I aim to shed some light on the intricate inner landscape, always hidden even from friends and family.

A painter's tool is his palette; my tools are my questions and listening. With terminal illness, you don't naturally see the existing light at the end of the tunnel. But it is in the very looking, the attention, that the true nature of existence is revealed. What life could be! What brightness it is! What fullness!

I began my research as a volunteer on the palliative care unit of the Royal Victoria Hospital in Montreal. I had heard about Jean Cameron, who had worked as a nurse at the same hospital and written *Time to Live, Time to Die,* a book about facing her terminal illness. I decided to take my questions to her and ask if they would be appropriate. By the time I reached her, she was already quite sick with cancer, which had slowly progressed over five years. When she heard my questions, her immediate response was, "I would like to answer those." I knew I was on the right track.

I thought my search for people to interview would be fairly straightforward. There were certainly plenty of dying people. I had meetings with doctors, nurses, social workers. I gave them a written proposal, talked to them, put out the call. Response was frustratingly slow. I met with many more health-care professionals than patients because, as I found out from my reading and volunteer work, most people with a terminal illness are in denial or are angry, terrified, or depressed.

Very slowly, names began to trickle in. Some of these people were appropriate interview subjects, some not. I found a newspaper article on Florence, who had ALS. A palliative care doctor suggested Norman.

Everyone who appears here recognized that talking would cleanse them, clarify certain issues, or give voice to recent realizations. All answered questions they had never been asked before, and many told me things they had never told anyone else for fear of not being understood.

Each interview was done one on one. I did not have to state that I didn't want anyone else present during the interviews. My subjects knew instinctively that they didn't want another person to hear what they would say. Neither of us wanted a third person, in front of whom my speakers might censor themselves. All the people I interviewed wanted to be free to talk. *They had a need to talk.*

After each interview, I would either transcribe the tapes or listen to them again and formulate more questions, based on what had been said, to take to the next meeting. I had to be very present to these people, hearing not just their words, but listening to and interpreting underlying feelings. Sometimes I missed the essence of what had been said, and it wasn't until I listened to the tapes at home that I fully understood the meaning of the words. Then, with greater understanding of the experiences recounted, I would formulate new questions for the next interview. I let my interviewees guide me more deeply into specific painful experiences to ascertain how these events might be connected to their present situation.

Since I wanted my subjects to be free to talk, I did ask them to tell me what names they preferred me to change and which incidents they would rather I not use. I automatically changed most names, but, with permission, I used the originals that were obviously appropriate. For example, in the case of Florence, it was ironic that she went to Florence to realize her ultimate dream and that her illness also began in that city.

I approached these people humbly, looking for answers that I was sure they had, even though they might be unaware of them. My line of questioning was individualized to suit the person. However, I did compile a list of questions that I asked at the final interview, when appropriate. Here are a few examples:

"Are we responsible for our lives? Are we responsible for our deaths?"

"Can the awareness of death refine the process of living?"

"Is there a right time to die?"

I believed everyone's story. I trusted them to tell me the truth; it was in their interest. These people had no reason to please or impress me. In many cases, body language spoke volumes about the authenticity of answers.

I conducted four to eight interviews with each person, the exception being Katherine, with whom I could do only two interviews. The second interview came just before Christmas, and she wanted to leave herself free for friends and family. Katherine was willing to continue after the holidays, but she was already quite sick, and she died before New Year's Day. With Sister Angela, I had only three meetings because she was too weak for any more; she died soon after our last meeting.

Each interview lasted two to four hours, and the total process often spanned several months. I then structured the resulting monologues cinematically, as if I were in a film editing room. I used about ten percent of the total interview material, using the 10:1 ratio that I normally worked with in film. In the end, I edited and structured all the interviews to bring coherence to each narrative, to highlight certain threads and themes.

I have included only three diseases in the book: cancer, AIDS, and ALS (amyotrophic lateral sclerosis), brought to public attention by the American baseball legend Lou Gehrig, who died from this disease in 1941, and now by Stephen Hawking, the physicist. ALS destroys the motor neurons in the brain and spinal cord which are responsible for sending messages to muscles throughout the body. As these neurons are destroyed, muscles atrophy and lose their ability to move. Eventually more and more muscles are affected, including those that control swallowing and breathing. Life expectancy is two to five years.

Both AIDS and ALS have societies that I contacted for potential names. There are innumerable types of cancers; Norman, Elaine, and Sister Angela all had different ones. My interest was not to cover a variety of diseases but to find ordinary people who, at a point of crisis, have reflected upon their lives. After lengthy research, these twelve people became my own random sample of humanity, as I found them, in Montreal at the end of the twentieth century.

I believe that reading these twelve portraits is like walking into a room with twelve strangers — some you will like, some you will not. Different people attract us at different times in our lives.

Everyone who appears in *A Good Enough Life* died within two weeks to nine months of the last interview, except Laura, who is still very much alive and active. Her portrait ends with a recurring dream she has had since the age of fifteen. In the dream she lives to be one hundred and four, yet today she has a terminal illness. Is it possible to overcome such odds?

Invariably, aspects of these lives will bring to mind details of one's own life experiences. I have added no commentary to these portraits. For me, as a writer, what is most important is that readers think, shape their own opinions, and reflect on what these people have revealed, what lessons have been learned. The purpose of this book is to stimulate you and spark questions. Though the questions may vary, certain answers will be universal. Particular patterns emerge from interview to interview, and I summarize these at the end of the book.

I am grateful to those who have participated in this venture. Their generosity has encouraged me to examine my own life, further explore certain questions, and formulate new ones. A most precious gift! May this book do the same for you.

"Upon one's death I wish people would remember the life, and it should be a good enough life that it puts a smile on a person's face."

— *Florence*

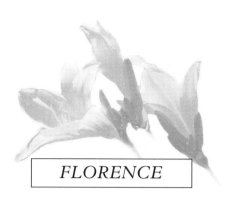

FLORENCE

Florence was a fifty-eight-year-old woman suffering from ALS. She was also a breast cancer survivor, so she had already faced death once before. She was the first person I interviewed. By the time I came to know her, I had met numerous terminally ill people who were either writing their own books or were not suitable informants. I had met no one who could help with my quest, who evoked my curiosity. I was losing hope of finding the kind of person I had in mind. Maybe I had it all wrong, maybe such people did not exist.

Then I came across an interesting article in the newspaper about Florence. She sounded intelligent, bright, ready to face her own death. I reasoned that, since she had already spoken to a journalist, she might be willing to speak to me. I called her. I told her some of the questions I would ask her. There would be several interviews. Yes, she consented. She had not asked for many details; I sensed an urgency to talk.

I showed up at her door for my first interview filled with anticipation and humility: to be terminally ill and to answer a stranger's probing questions would not be easy for her. I was surprised to find that she was more than willing to talk, an opportunity which did not come her way too often. Over time, I found that the interviews gave her a chance to put her thoughts into words. My questions made her think deeper.

She welcomed me into her house with a warm smile, wearing a sweatsuit and leaning on a walker. She was about five foot two, round, with brown hair. She pointed me toward her living room, which was littered with The New York Times. *The book review section was open. We sat down on the couch and began to talk. The rapport was immediate. We had read the same books, had common reference points, plus her parents had been Italian. I told her I had written a book about an Italian family. She wanted to read it and asked me to bring a copy to the next interview.*

As her story unfolded and as I fed her more and more questions, I could tell she was making connections that she had not made before. At the end of the last interview, as we said goodbye, there was ambivalence about whether we should keep in touch. I telephoned her a few times to talk about a good book review, an interesting book. During one of our telephone conversations, slightly hesitant, uncertain whether I should be asking her this question since, after all, she was dying, I wondered aloud if she would like me to visit her. She said that this was now a time for her to be alone or with her family. I appreciated her honesty.

Dying is a learning process. Right now I'm trying to learn how to be a fairly decent model for my children, a model of someone leaving this life. But I don't know what that means. I don't want to be an embarrassment. Yet I embarrass myself constantly. I start laughing at a joke and find it very hard to stop. I cry at the smallest sad thought that goes through my mind. If I'm in an emotional state, I find it very difficult to speak, my words get slurred. I wet my pants. I don't know how one handles this in the right and proper way. A model for young people is where you can admire someone's acts. Well, all my acts now are foolish and weak.

I wanted to grow up to be strong like my grandmother, who to me was a mountain of strength. All the women in my family have been strong. And I always appreciated strength in myself, the ability to take control, be in charge. "Do you need something done? Do you feel confused? Come to me, I'll do it."

Now I drop a stamp and say, "Brian, will you please pick up the stamp?"

I never liked that. The kind of woman who has things done for her was not the kind of woman I emulated. And since the illness, I'm no longer a strong woman. Watching my strength diminish has been very hard and has been accompanied by tremendous guilt. I can't get out of a chair alone. I can no longer do some very basic things. I need to ask for help, and that's always been hard for me.

As a child I was so painfully shy. And the period between thirteen and seventeen was a very lonely and uncomfortable time in which I gritted my teeth and decided to change things. I went to a strict Catholic girls' high school and just made myself do glee club and solos. I made myself get into the honours society. And it was all so painful. Yet overcoming my shyness gave me a strong feeling of success.

But I think I have acted out of fear very often. Fear has been my great vice. When I was in college studying music, I had a wonderful voice teacher who taught many famous singers. She offered to put me in the course at the Met.

My father said, "You do that and I will never support you."

This was an overwhelming statement. I had worked part-time since I was fifteen and had given all my money to my parents. I had won three university scholarships, so I didn't need money for school. I knew how to earn money, yet when my father said, "I will never support you again," I thought I was falling through the earth. So I stopped thinking about a career in music and did as my father wanted. I got my teaching licences both for the state and the city of New York. It seemed so prudent, steady, and sure-thinking to get my teacher's licence. He said it would be something I could always fall back on. But I just didn't enjoy teaching. I had learned to teach out of fear.

After my children were in school, when I wanted to fall back on those teaching licences, there was no need for teachers. There was a glut of teachers. Suddenly I realized the irony of it and started to think of those performances I had missed at the Metropolitan Opera and all those singers I didn't hear. It would have been a magical time taking courses at the Met, even if it would have lasted only a year or two. So I told all my children to do what they loved. Now Martin, who is twenty-six, is a teacher and teaches all over the globe because he loves to travel. Jerry, who is twenty-eight, makes films. Stella, who is twenty-nine, is a painter, and Pamela, who is thirty, is the steady one. I think she has acquired my fearful, careful disposition because she has a very good job. She studied piano till she got her degree, then became a physiotherapist. Now she's doing her master's, and that's the kind of life I led, and I think we both live our lives with a measure of fear.

Though I say fear has been my vice, I have also always felt you must live so that when you die you don't regret all the things you didn't do. I suppose the only regret I have is not singing at the Met. I should have done it.

If I could change anything in my life, I would change my relationship to my mother. I was very fortunate to have my grandmother. My mother and I tried to get along, but we usually fought. I've been a very critical person and criticized my mother even if I never said anything. I'm sure she knew I didn't approve of her. Even when she was dying in the hospital, I was being critical of her. She was angry because she couldn't solve a mundane problem. And it seemed to me she was wasting good time that should be used praying, finding solace in God. It's not that I think everyone should have a deathbed conversion. But my mother had been very religious, and once she even had a vision of Jesus. About a month after my father's death, she was lying down and Jesus appeared at the foot of her bed. This had made her very happy.

So here is a woman who once had a vision of Jesus, and she's arguing with someone over property, struggling over a piece of land. What does it mean at this point? You could be having another vision. I said to her in hospital, "That piece of land is not really your home, your home is with Jesus."

She looked at me and said, "Are you making fun of me?"

And I thought, Oh my God, is that what I sound like?

I didn't know what to do or say after that. And I was frantic that she was going to die with a frown on her face.

A few days later, I went out for lunch, and when I came back my mother was dead. In death she had the face of a doll. There was just emptiness, nothing, nada, gone. An empty doll's face. It was such a gigantic cancellation. It strikes you with such power that you can't imagine anything going on anymore. I think with every dead person I've seen there has been a loss of faith, because there is nothing so utterly gone and finished as a corpse.

When my mother died, my great regret was that I could not cry. All the grandchildren cried, but none of her three children cried. Yet when I was seventeen and my grandmother died, I cried, I screamed, threw myself on the sofa, it was a real drama. But I couldn't grieve my mother's death.

Now, every once in a while, I think back to my life and try to judge if I've used it well or well enough, but I suppose no one ever uses their life well enough. I have not exactly been a workaholic. I have enjoyed my life, relaxed, wasted time. Sometimes you regret the relaxation, the fun. You think, maybe I could have been more of a scholar. Now I do more than relax, I do nothing at all. And doing nothing at all is very valuable, it can be extremely creative. In fact, you really can't do anything creative unless you do nothing at all periodically. And doing nothing at all, letting go, is a state of prayer. It's very hard to do that.

When I was a chaplain at McGill University, I was interested in prayer, and I used to read all kinds of books about prayer, and there were lots of students also reading all kinds of books about prayer and asking me for the latest edition. And reading is not praying. But there's always another book you need to read first. It's much easier to be busy. I know, because I have always been a doer.

Before, when I was well, I led an active life. I ran around. It's so easy to live on the surface of life, there are constant distractions. Now that I can hardly move from one room to the next, and soon I'll need help to go to the bathroom, I'm learning that there is great wisdom in silence. These days especially, it's very, very important for me to pray every day. At least once a day I go into my room to meditate, and I haven't done this in years. And I have time to think about my life.

After my mother's death, I realized she had fulfilled my wildest dreams. What irony! When I learned about my inheritance, I thought, I don't want to fritter this money away the way I usually do. I want to do something. What is the thing you want most in the world? To my great surprise, I wanted to be in a monastery in Italy to finish my book. It was a totally self-indulgent wish, and I gave it to myself, with the help of my mother.

I had wanted to go to Europe for a long time. When I was young, I even saved up enough money to go and then didn't. This happened a few times, and of course there was a reason for it. My parents were supposed to go to Europe for their honeymoon, but my father had an automobile accident and there was no trip. So my mother said none of us were going to Europe before she did. That held me back, but also I think I was afraid of being on my own in a strange country.

My mother never did go to Europe. Then she dies and leaves me an inheritance. And I go not just to Europe, I go to Italy, straight to Florence. I decided that was my spiritual home. I was going to break out of this north/south conflict and go right in the middle.

When I was young, I used to beg my grandmother to tell me about her past, about Italy. She would tell me nothing. "It is all finished," she said. My aunt said something similar once: "Don't look back. You have to live and look forward."

That was something my grandmother had passed on to her daughters. I knew she had been born in Genoa, and for a while she lived in Argentina, and then at the age of seventeen she crossed the ocean all by herself, came to New York, got a job, and worked till she met my grandfather. What fired her up to do such a thing at the turn of the century? Why all this travelling at such a young age? I asked my aunts and uncles about my grandmother's past, and no one knew any more than I did.

My grandmother spoke a little broken English. My mother spoke a little broken Italian. So my mother and grandmother didn't even speak the same language. My grandmother had very solid, old-fashioned beliefs, and my mother hated to cook. She was the frozen-food girl. My mother and my aunt were beauty contest winners. They were flappers, Charleston girls, and they put anything Italian as far away from them as they could. They belonged to America. My grandmother's world was friends, food, the community of Italian immigrants, the church, and, of course, the family first and foremost. When I was young, every Sunday of my life was spent around my grandmother's table from about eleven in the morning to four in the afternoon.

Maybe my mother didn't completely reject her mother's world because, when it came time to marry, my grandmother picked out a boy for her, and she accepted. My father was also Italian, the first generation to be born in New York, like my mother. Maybe I was the complete rejector. I married someone Irish. When my father came around with Italian young men, I served them an aperitif and left the room. I would not have anything to do with them.

Then, at the age of fifty-four, I go to Italy to learn Italian, the language my mother had disdained like everything Italian. I went as soon as I got the inheritance, about a year after my mother's death. And it changed my life. When you give yourself the ultimate gift you desire, then you can never again be envious of anyone else. Up until then, my life was mostly duty, and the trip to Florence was frivolity. It was a marvellous cure for all the nasty feelings I had. I was envious of others because I didn't see myself as having fun. I did all the dutiful things, which breeds resentment. I was someone who worked hard. And I wanted to think in terms of fun.

Originally my son was going to go to Florence to take a two-week course in Italian. He decided not to go. When he learned that I planned to go instead, he said, "Don't go for only two weeks, go for a month."

I thought it seemed so daring. Then I thought, Why go for only a month?

And it grew. Christmas was a natural barrier. I wanted to be back here with my family for Christmas, which gave me nearly four months in Florence.

For the first month I stayed in a British guest house, taking Italian every day, going to museums, seeing the city, eating gelati. It was wonderful. After a month, I moved to a monastery for the rest of the time to work on my book, which is about the search for beauty and the effect of beauty on our lives. Is beauty divine? Can beauty redeem our human poverty? Can it redeem death? It started as a Ph.D. thesis without footnotes. Before I began working on it, I asked myself the same question I was to ask when I got the inheritance: What do I want to write about more than anything else in the world?

Wanting to write this book was like wanting to sing at the Met. This is a work of art that is completely unjustified. It's not a part of duty. It's for my pleasure. Writing it is like a spiritual quest. Maybe it's a thing I must do to save my soul. It's not practical in terms of materialism.

The book is based on my own experiences from 1989 to 1994. The key question was, can beauty lead one to God? The question grew out of something Camus had written about a terrible sadness that accompanies the experience of true beauty. If beauty is so wonderful, why does it make us feel so terribly sad? You apprehend beauty, and it almost strikes your heart in two. You see beauty, and you can't hold it in your hands. You can't put it in your pocket and take it home, it's other. It doesn't belong to you. And God is other, you can never contain or define it. So beauty is your first experience of transcendence. It sets up an appetite, a yearning. And I think that yearning can eventually lead one to love and to God.

My illness began in November, at the monastery, while I was ful-filling my ultimate desire in Florence. One day I came down with a fever. And that night I had a dream that a horde of cats had broken in through the basement window. There was a screen on the window, and the cats just pushed it in and commandeered my house. I didn't take it as a good dream. To me it meant that something had flooded me, something had taken over. I woke up with a fever and cramps in my legs, and when I got up to walk, my knees were stiff.

Though the fever went away, the stiffness and cramps continued, and added to that was a weakness in my right ankle, so that my ankle would give way unexpectedly, and I was afraid of tripping. I wrote all this down in my journal. The fever lasted about three days, but ten days later I'm writing about my stiff knees reminding me of my rusty typewriter. It was so humid, it was raining constantly, and my room was full of green mould. It was growing all over the walls, and eventually I had to throw away my typewriter because it got so rusty. That's how wet it was. I blamed everything on the damp weather.

However, when I left the bad weather and came back to Montreal in December, the symptoms continued, though they didn't develop in severity till the following summer. And that's when I saw a doctor.

After I was diagnosed with ALS in September, I felt embarrassed to ask my doctor about how much longer I had left to live. I did write a letter asking him to tell me how much time he thought I had. When I later saw him, he seemed very sad, and I never did get an answer to my question. It's been hard to talk about this. I'm more comfortable asking someone like the occupational therapist, who is like a girl-friend. She said she had one patient who lasted nine months, and another patient lasted five years, but she was in very good condition to begin with, and that was very rare. She said the average seems to be two years. The physios have told me what to expect. The doctor didn't tell me much, but I know how the disease progresses. I've read booklets about it.

In the beginning the illness was surrounded by guilt. Then, as my body diminished, I got extremely angry. Angry and fearful. Though the disease affects motor control, it doesn't affect intelligence. The brain cells that control the conscious motor activities, like lifting up a book, are dying. But also I seem to have no control over my emotions. This is terribly embarrassing. I laugh at the stupidest joke and cannot stop. And the voice that's laughing is not my own anymore. The voice I'm speaking with now is kind of hoarse, and when I laugh it gets even deeper and I don't feel like myself. I think I must sound bizarre, silly. I have to explain to my friends or family that to laugh at the slightest provocation or weep uncontrollable sobs over the smallest things is part of the disease. There are muscles in my face that no longer work. So a smile becomes a guffaw, a sad feeling becomes a sob. I become absolutely transparent. I cannot hide my feelings from others. Sometimes I feel very happy to see somebody and I'll cry or laugh. I never know when I'm going to fall on my face, figuratively or literally. At the beginning of the winter I used to be able to walk with a cane. Now I need a walker. Next it will be a wheelchair. I'm worried about being alone because I'm going to fall. Now I can barely use my hands. I need a special knife to cut my meat. In a period of sometimes only weeks, I see degeneration. It seems to be happening very fast.

But if you relax and don't keep trying to do the old things, you experience life in a new way. Once I discovered I didn't have to dress, wash, and make my breakfast for me or anyone else, and I didn't have to be ashamed about not doing that, I could really enjoy watching someone else — apparently enjoying him or herself — making me a meal. They seem happy and I'm in a state of adoration. I would never have allowed this to happen willingly. Now it's happening and I'm enjoying it. I don't have to feel guilty about it.

My illness has brought such wonderful things out of the children and Brian. It brings out the best in most people, but I don't know if it brings out the best in me because I'm the centre of attention and people take care of me. There's been nothing to test me to see where the best of me is. I haven't been challenged to do anything. The challenge is simply to receive and to accept. At first that was difficult, and now I find that receiving and accepting is a very easy and nice thing to do. Now I don't have to make the great dinner and impress people with the way I can cook because they do it for me. I don't have to write the great paper and impress people with how smart I am because my children are writing papers, and they give them to me to read, and I enjoy that very much. I'm no longer striving to be the centre of attention, but I am anyway.

So the illness is not all diminishment, it's also a gain, a new kind of knowledge. Since the diagnosis, there have been discoveries of the value of friendship, family, courtesy, and a good sense of humour. It's not anything new, but a discovery on a deeper level. I guess you're always learning the same things over and over but on a deeper level.

I think it's all part of a necessary preparation when approaching death. In the beginning, it's hard to think that you're preparing for death because you want to think about life. Even if you want to think about death, you feel guilty because that's like giving up, and you're very much encouraged to think about life. Or you don't think about it because you're afraid. But I think it's essential to prepare for death.

This is the second time I'm preparing for death. The first time was nine years ago, when I had cancer. I went into analysis then because I needed to really study my life. I had a tremendous desire for understanding my choices, why things fell apart, and what do I want to do differently. Though at the time I was saying, I want to understand my life because I want to know how to change the way I'm living, now I see it was really a preparation for death.

Of course, there is the practical part, too. You prepare the will, the funeral, but you're also saying, I'm going through this process and people are observing me and what are they seeing? They're sometimes seeing a very goofy person who pees in her pants when she laughs too much and has to change her clothes in the middle of a party. And then you think, Is that what I really want them to remember about me?

Dying is a learning process. I've never done it before, so every step is new. I'm learning something new about my body, my methods of coping, my abilities, my disabilities, learning about how other people react to my sudden weakness, my sudden silliness. Sometimes I'm very, very silly. I'm no longer the person I was. I'm no longer the person with the armour, the persona everyone has grown used to. I'm completely different, and that has required a lot of changes from people around me.

I'm very aware of losing my ability to speak because I used to sing at parties and in concerts. I won my husband through singing Irish ballads. He always saw me as a singer. Brian married the girl who sang Irish songs. Now I listen.

These days I have a real problem talking, but there is no problem when I'm asleep. In my dreams, not only am I talking, I'm singing very well. And I love it. I also walk easily in my dreams, and I'm surprised. I think to myself, Why don't I do this all the time? Maybe I'm afraid and only doing this to myself. Maybe I've gotten into the habit of not walking.

In my dream, I'm not sick, so it seems I'm hung up on something that makes it hard for me to walk in real life. This has happened a few times. It does give you a double life.

All my children have dreams of flying, whereas I've flown only once in a dream. When I was about three or four years old, I dreamt that I was flying an aeroplane but I didn't know how, so I crashed into my grandmother's grape arbour that she had in the back yard. Crashing ended my flying career. And even then I wasn't flying myself, I didn't know how to fly. It was about not being able to control your life. All these adults telling you what to do.

These days I feel as if I've gone back to childhood again. I'm being touched as much as when I was an infant. I'm glorying in the sense of touch, and that's extremely nice. Also, I'm finding the utmost delight in simple, old-fashioned dishes. I desire simple foods like meat loaf, Jell-O. They taste so good that I can laugh. It's no longer, I'll make you an osso bucco you'll never forget. Now give me a good baked potato and I'll be very, very happy. I don't know if that's an improvement or a diminishment of taste buds.

Before, I tended to have a jaded, fussy palate, and this can be viewed as a reflection of one's appetite for life as well. One desires more and more special experiences. One wants to travel to exotic cities, taste exotic foods. One is always looking for change, trying to top the last event. I had a very big appetite for life, for everything, for all cultures. Now I'm just so glad I can eat and it doesn't upset my stomach. By necessity I've narrowed my priorities. It's like a distillation. I have a hunger to attend to basic relationships and basic ideas. But if I were in great pain, I think I would be cranky and self-centred, and I would annoy everyone till they gave me something to take the pain away. I'm very, very grateful not to have to deal with pain. I have this luxury of indulging my thoughts and asking questions.

My public question was, if I'm faced with pain and uselessness, do I go along with the very common-sense and compassionate idea of doctor-assisted suicide? And I surprised myself by saying no. Of course, I don't know if I'm going to change my mind. But right now I say no because I feel there is something to be gained every inch of the way, something new to be learned. As questions come up and you search for answers, you're learning more about yourself and life, maybe more than ever before because the questions are more urgent. This might be the last time I get a chance to find an answer to this question, so I better be serious about it.

I'm learning how to live in a receptive mode as opposed to an active mode because I have no choice. Before, when I had a choice, I did what suited me, and usually it feels much better to have control and get what you want when you want it. And this modern part of me is being taken away.

In the past I have taken control of things because I felt people couldn't make decisions on their own, and I'm not patient enough to wait, so I just get them to do this or that. Or I'm going to do this or that for them because I know it's right. I've lived much of my life like that. Choice, power, action, all those things we value in Western civilization, I'm losing. Now the illness is teaching me that if I can't do anything, if I can only receive, I'm still learning and I'm still living a valuable life. Though it's not necessarily the life of the Western world.

I'm beginning to see that what we learn doesn't have to shine out. Learning is not invalidated when it's private. You're still learning, growing, even if it's interior and you're not establishing a new religion, a new university, you're just growing inside yourself. It would be nice to think that that had an effect on others. Maybe it does.

Internal growth should be encouraged, validated even though it doesn't have the external rewards of power and success. Our society tends to diminish the value of interiority. The inner life is suspect. You have to be sociable, practical, dependable, and if you keep to yourself, there's something wrong with you. We undervalue solitude, silence, and interior growth because we don't see it.

I remember having an argument about losing yourself or finding yourself with a doctor friend. I was saying what a wonderful experience it was to lose yourself, and she said, "You mean, find yourself." And we just couldn't understand one another. Someone said you find yourself when you lose yourself. Maybe that's it. Did I lose myself when I went to Florence? Did I lose myself with this illness? Or did I really find myself?

The biggest surprise of my life was seeing Brian come back, move in, squeeze my orange juice, and make my breakfast in the mornings. I wouldn't have believed that could ever happen. We separated ten years ago and only kept in touch through the children. And Brian had a five-year relationship with another woman. This was nothing I ever expected would change. Yet he's come back to be with me and told me that the relationship is over. Brian does have a very highly developed sense of duty, and I guess he felt he had to make a choice between her and me. He has given up a comfortable life to be here with me in a crowded space, sleeping on a sofa. And I've just been so happily surprised because Brian has never been this wonderful. He wakes me in the morning with a joke and a kiss, bathes me and dresses me. He shops for me, takes me to appointments, to the homes of friends. He allows me to continue living as normally as possible. Otherwise, I would be confined to a nursing home now. And we're very happy. Very often he says that he's surprised how happy he is and how well his work is going. Brian is again with the family, and that makes him feel secure about who he is. He had wanted very much to see the kids more often, and they're here almost all the time. He feels he has returned to a certain course or image of himself that he likes very much.

I think Brian had wanted a sabbatical from marriage. And he did it even though I loved him and he still loved me. The year before the separation, I knew he wanted to leave, but he didn't want to leave. This was a few years after we had arrived in Montreal. We had moved from New York to Montreal when Brian got a position teaching engineering at McGill University. At that time, he said, "You can study whatever you want."

I enrolled at McGill and got my Bachelor of Theology and was working on my Master's in Religious Studies when I was hired to be a chaplain at McGill. So, pretty well from the moment we arrived, we were each preoccupied with our own goals and trying to fit into our environment. It took us a few years to settle in, set down roots, get our bearings. Six years later, it seemed we were heading in different directions. And we began to argue. The arguments were wearing me down. For instance, there would be an argument after Thursday night dinner, and I'd say, "If you want to go out, if you want to see someone, you don't have to pick a fight over it."

And he would say, "Of course I'm not seeing anyone. You just make dinner too late."

Then at a certain point he said, "I still feel young, and I want to have some fun."

But our arguments were about dinner being too late or I spent too much on groceries. I felt terrible. I felt worse than I ever felt in my life. So, after a year of arguing, when he actually left, I helped him move because it was such a relief to stop the fighting.

The separation happened when the kids were teenagers and just beginning to date, so this affected their attitude toward relationships in that they didn't trust them to last. But if you understand that marriage is a process of learning about yourself and someone else, it's a kind of school where you both continue to develop, I think that's helpful. We break up because we're so threatened and we're so hurt.

Six months after Brian left, I felt a pea-sized lump in my breast. It was a malignant cancer that hadn't spread yet, so I was very lucky. I'm sure this was a stress cancer, probably because I didn't want to talk about how I was feeling to anybody. Even after I found out I had breast cancer, I didn't let anyone see me cry. My daughter Stella complained about it and was sad. My daughter Pam was angry. I didn't express these feelings, I think they expressed them for me.

After the operation I had chemotherapy. Every morning I spent at the Montreal General, in the chemotherapy waiting room with other people. We all had our bodies marked in different places with a red Magic Marker. It was another world, a world within a world. I felt we were now in a separate place that most people didn't know about. It was the world of the sick, the world of the cancer patient, and it was completely other.

I decided to go into analysis and think about what had brought me here. I had come to a dead end. It was just before my fiftieth birthday. I had lost my family. I had lost my career. I had left the chaplaincy and the Church. And I had nearly lost my life. I was obviously not doing very well leading my own ship.

In the past, when I had a spiritual problem, I spoke to a priest. But at this point in my life the priests were the enemies. The priests were saying that we women were celebrating a Black Mass, and there was no way that I could turn to a priest. And I felt I needed to talk to someone.

The most important realization of analysis was that I was highly inflated. I felt I had been working to change the Church and God was behind this. To think such things just overwhelms the ego. After that I came to be very weary of the global feelings you are filled with when you are part of a group. So I left the Church, the feminist movement, socialism, and I tried very deliberately to strip myself of all group mentalities to see if there was anything left. I hoped I would find my own voice, my own soul.

I thought leaving the group voices behind would be like peeling off the layers of the onion, and in the middle I would find the pearl of great value, something firm, well shaped, clearly defined, a hard crystal of identity. And I didn't find anything. Just emptiness. I then fashioned this into the idea of receptivity, like you have an empty room, a guest room, into which an idea or person or some spirit might enter. I made a good thing of it. But I believe other people do have something very firm and clearly defined because they seem so sure of their ideas, so sure about where they're going and what they believe, and they tell others about it as if it were an absolute truth, a fundamental given, certain that others will benefit. I don't have anything that strong that I can say.

Within me there is always a voice questioning any absolute statement I might make. I do believe that humankind is born with the knowledge that to kill another is evil. And then a little voice will say, All the time?

I don't know if I believe in absolutes anymore. For me, personally, there is God, and I would call God the essence of love. I would describe it as a very loving presence that I feel at certain very fortunate times. But I would never dream of setting out to prove this to anyone else.

Neither do I want to say I believe in absolute evil as opposed to absolute love. I find that evil is very subtle, and it's interwoven in my life. The basis of evil is withholding affection, and once you're withholding, just think of the things you can do to the other person. You can commit atrocities. I can. I'm not always aware of when I'm hurting or harming till after the words have come out of my mouth and I realize I've hurt this person. Then I ask myself, Why have I said this? I perceive in the doing that this was not the right thing to do or say, and I question my motives. Usually it's a disinclination to care. The motive between an evil word or a kind word is a lack of love. That's evil because, I think, we have an unwritten contract to look out for one another. And sometimes I just couldn't care less, and I withhold or I'm abrupt. If you become used to withholding, you begin to act in callous ways.

Of course, you can also withhold out of self-protection, and real self-protection is not evil. We need to protect ourselves. I don't think you can be open and giving to everyone all the time. It's all situational.

For instance, around the time Brian left and I realized I had breast cancer, I was withholding from my children by not talking to them. I was presenting a strong front that was false. Yes, I was protecting myself, but I was also withholding, which caused them emotional difficulties. But for me that was a time of disillusionment and a shedding of a way of life. I was in the process of leaving the Church.

Catholicism had been so much a part of my life. When I was seventeen I decided I was going to be a nun, a little sister of the poor. I was trying to fill out the application form in my bedroom, which I shared with my sister, and it was one of those rare moments of being alone. There was a questionnaire attached to the form which asked, among other things, if I was legitimate, if I drank or smoked. I was deeply disturbed. I wouldn't even ask my mother some of this. Then I started thinking negatively: nuns have to wear black robes all the time, and they're not allowed to go out unless chaperoned, while I've seen priests in their plaid flannel shirts playing golf. And I was radicalized. I wanted to be a priest. Why should I be a nun? But I was also very frightened of making the decision not to be a nun because I believed in Satan. I felt absolute evil as a malevolent presence, as God is a benevolent presence. I felt that if I wanted to invite this malevolent presence in, I could. And I felt I must not even think about it. I felt on the borderline between good and evil because I saw it in those terms. But I didn't want any part in an exclusive group of nuns. And I said something very romantic like, I cast my lot with the mob. Or the masses.

I must have been pretty overwhelmed by this statement because I had an experience of levitation. I felt myself about three feet up in the air, over the bed. And I was scared. It was the first and last time that ever happened to me.

When I was up there, suspended, I made a choice, a choice for secularity, not to be part of Holy Mother Church, not to be a privileged virgin, but to be ordinary with no special privileges. And this very resonant male voice, like a radio voice, said, "You are barred from hell, but . . ." Once on the bed again, I completely forgot the words after "but." But what? But what? For years the most horrible thing I could think of was that "but . . . ." Much later I finally realized what it was: BUT you're going to lose your faith.

After I was married and already had the four children, NBC came and interviewed some people at my church in New Jersey, at St. Mary's, and I said on TV that I wanted to be a priest. Finally, it was out in public. To me, being ordained as a priest meant you had reached adulthood. At around that time Brian was invited to come to Montreal to teach at McGill, and I decided I wanted to study religion. Obviously I would need some background if I was going to become a priest. The director of the chaplaincy at the university was a priest. A few years after being at McGill, I went over to see him one day and said, "Who's your woman? Who do you work with?"

He didn't have a woman on his staff. He was a young man, very open, so he invited me to join him, and I became a chaplain. I preached on Sunday, I was available to students, I gave premarital courses. I was a chaplain for Dignity, which is a Catholic gay group.

During this time, I had many women friends who were eager to get together and pray. So we decided to hold our own women's Mass. Each month we went to a different house. The person whose house it was at also presided. We consecrated our own Mass with our own words, and it was always different. Several times I led the group and prayed to the goddess. At first I found that very difficult but after a while I learned to pray to Greek deities and goddesses. As I found aspects of the Pantheon that related to my life and needs, I began to see monotheism as cramping because monotheistic thought led to seeing things in black and white, led to pronouncements of good and evil, and was really a very fundamentalist way of thinking. I was drawn to polytheism and could see Krishna and Jesus as different manifestations of one God.

During the three years that our women's Mass lasted, I found our liturgies and meeting the women in this way very beautiful. To hear someone else pray is more intimate than physical touch. But gradually terrible rumours began to spread among the Catholics, saying we were a group of witches holding a Black Mass.

Originally I became a chaplain as a critic. I entered the Church with the idea of reformation. I was going to help bring the Church into the modern world. What wild dreams I had! I felt that my way of showing love to the Church was to be very vocal and try to change it. And I wasn't all that appreciated.

I complained to the president of the Paulist order, an American order of priests that sent directors up to the Newman Centre at McGill. They were not interested in listening. I continued to complain, and finally they sent up a new director who didn't even want to talk to me. This new director arrived the very same day that Brian moved out of the house. I went to the airport to meet him, and he paid absolutely no attention to me, as if I didn't exist.

The year-long argument with Brian had just ended with our separation, and now here comes this new director, and I just couldn't start arguing with him. I was too tired. So I avoided confrontations. Still, things were not going well because we weren't even talking to one another. I had worked there for five years before he came, and I felt we had achieved a lot, and he wasn't interested. So I offered my resignation. I left totally drained, disillusioned. I learned that you could change the Church cosmetically, you can have very nice discussions, but you come to a point where you hit a stone wall. The Church was like a totalitarian dictatorship, it had gone in the direction of Empire and Establishment.

Also, since the Catholic Church was for men, I didn't belong in it. If women are not permitted to be ordained as priests because Christ was a man and Christ didn't ordain women, then that meant this was a men's Church and Christ is obviously a man's God. The image of Christ or God that we've been taught was within us I don't have because I'm not a man. So at a time when I really needed God the most, after I had lost my marriage and my career, I just refused to turn to Him because it would have been dishonest. All the things that had comforted me or given me strength were not mine any longer. For me that was tremendously profound. It hit at the core of my being.

My last night at the Newman Centre was Christmas Eve. I preached the midnight service and never went back.

In January I started my doctoral work in religious studies, and on February 4 I had my breast cancer operation. It was very sudden. After the operation, I continued my doctoral work and returned to chaplaincy, but this time with the Anglicans.

For a time I worked as a chaplain at an AIDS hospice. I did everything there, I cleaned toilets, changed diapers, urine bags. We all did everything. I thought, this is like the *Catholic Worker*. There is no hierarchy here. I love this. What I discovered was that there is always a hierarchy, it just goes undercover. What we had there was a hierarchy of information. We were all supposed to be equal, but not everyone knew everything about what was going on. And, of course, not everyone had a say.

Still, the hospice gave me a lot. I had wonderful relationships with many of the patients, especially one, Matthew. My experiences with him triggered the idea for my book. He was such a case. He would say, "I'm a case, I'm a pillow case." He had been thrown out of the hospital because he was insane in many ways. He had everything wrong with him and arrived on a stretcher, bedridden, spitting, and cursing at people. He lived three of the four months I was there, and those three months were a lifetime for him. He changed radically. He was a miracle. And he made my life there so very rich. I called him my teacher. He taught me how to communicate without words and without rationality. He could read my mind, my moods. He would slip under my skin. He would talk as if he were me and the boundaries just slipped.

Matthew had been a hairdresser, a colourist, with very high standards of beauty, and he could just destroy a woman. There were volunteers who ran into him and never came back. His idea of feminine beauty was someone as thin as himself, and he was very thin. Though he loved beauty as I did, for him it seemed to get in the way of love. For him, beauty was an obstacle because he saw the surface right away and if it didn't please him he'd curse you.

I had to learn how to talk to him. It wasn't always rational, it was more like picking up on intuitions and I loved it. It just expanded possibilities for me. I was prepared to try to make sense out of his nonsense, something that was hard for me to do because of my rigidity. It really stretched me. When I got into the idea of play, of being able to just play and be silly and let the words flow, then it happened. He also taught me to be bawdy. He had such a dirty mouth but we were all laughing. Being with him showed me the value of imagination, play, and truthfulness.

At the hospice, he recognized and experienced love. Physically he got better and better. He was actually reading. And he became very content. He didn't stop using foul language, but he would curse in a happy way instead of a nasty way.

Then he became an inconvenience because he was living too long.

And it was decided that he needed to prepare for death. I was very angry when I heard this. I expressed the anger at a staff meeting and was told, "Florence, everyone has to die. Death isn't such a terrible thing. What did you expect?"

I tried to tell them that we have to respect the patient's own timing. I didn't think it was right to force it on him. It was presented back to me that I had a problem with death. The next day, someone told him he was going to die, and he better start thinking about it. He started to cry and got depressed. From then on he went downhill, and very soon he died.

I left the hospice. Two years later, my mother died and left an inheritance giving me the time to work on the book Matthew had inspired.

During the four months I was at the AIDS hospice, there were eight deaths. The people always waited to die until after I had left, very often fifteen minutes after I had left.

Before my father died, he told my mother to go to church. She had been gone no more than forty minutes, and when she came back he was dead. I believe that death is a private act. It is the most private act, the most secret garden.

I think when people die they want to be alone because all the people you love are standing around you, and you're clinging to them. They keep you alive, they keep you desiring to live. But if you're at the point of death, you would really be much happier if they left you alone because you need to focus away from life. You must be able to let go and give yourself over to this dark mystery. You must turn away from those you love and face into the darkness. And I believe that love calls us into the darkness. Transcendent love. I don't think I'd want other people in my room at that very moment of death because it will be between me and God. If this is the moment to meet God, then it's the moment to meet God. In a way all of life is a building up to a certain moment of revelation.

Preparing for death happens on many levels, and the first and obvious one is the practical level. How to dispose of the things you own? How to provide for the business of being buried?

The next level is a spiritual preparation for death. That's ongoing. You prepare so much, and then you probably have to undergo a sudden suffering, be it physical or emotional, and you continue to prepare from that next level. For me, one cause of suffering is seeing myself lose capacities. Each time there is something new, I must face it, come to terms with it, and continue on. I think that suffering is just a deepening that also has to do with character reformation. As we die, we have to work on the knots and kinks we've made in our character. It's a matter of purifying ourselves. As we do this, we become more spiritual, come closer to God.

The dark side of this illness is sorrow over eventual parting. There is the sadness of leaving people. None of my children are married yet, and none of them have children. I'd love to go to the weddings. I'd love to play with the babies, my grandchildren, I'd love to see them grow, and I won't be able to do that. Thinking of this, I may suddenly cry, and it may go just as quickly.

But if you are living vitally, it is not so hard to die. It's hardest to die when you haven't done anything. It's painful to die if you haven't lived. Is it possible to live yet be ready for death? It's part of the philosophy of, do what you want now. Like they write in greeting cards, tell people you love them now. Don't reserve presents for birthdays. If you feel like giving a present, give it now. I think I've tried to live like that. And if you try to live like that, you're kind of up-to-date and you're ready. But I desire more and more loving and giving and enjoying and laughing. I desire this so much that it makes me cry to think it'll end. But at the same time I'm ready to go when the time comes.

I'm seeing the children's sadness and I don't know what to do about that. One of my daughters is under great stress, and apparently I'm the major cause of it. She worries about me all the time. I try to make her see that I'm okay, but it doesn't help. My illness is a problem. I'm trying to find ways to lower the threatening feeling she has. It's something I'm working on, day to day. It's something she has to work out, too. I said something terrible to her the other day. I said, "If you're feeling so bad now, how are you going to feel when I die?"

I know that was cruel, but I felt I had to say it. The more we keep

reality before us, the easier it will be to let go. But I think it's easier
to let go for the dying than for the living because eventually the dying
person becomes very tired. That's what I've seen. Over time, in preparation for death, one gradually lets go of the interests and activities
that had once been important. The living must go on without you.

I do want to talk about it. I don't want dying to be something we
never mention. If you hide it and pretend it's not there and suddenly
it's there, I think the letting go will be more difficult in the end. I'm
trying to figure it out. It's the first time I've done this. It does seem
best to talk about it. I have mentioned it in passing, but to have a
deep conversation about death with everyone in the family seems like
a biggie.

I don't usually think about death. You don't know how it's going
to be until it's over. You can only go from day to day. But the other
day something strange happened. I suddenly felt a chill, and I got the
afghan from the sofa and I just wrapped it around me. But I couldn't
get warm. I was so cold, and I started to cry. At that moment I was
afraid of death. I had a terrible chill and I couldn't get warm and I
cried. It lasted ten minutes. It seemed like a long time. So there are
times of panic.

The feeling of fear comes and goes, the fear that I'm really sick,
it's going to get worse, and how long will it take. I don't want to
suffer. I've read there are saints who have been purified by suffering,
purified of all the dross, all the frailties and failures, envies and
resentments, and they became pure burning coals of love. Well, I
have never known people like that. What I know about suffering is
that it diminishes you. From my experience, suffering confines you to
your body. Your body with all its aches and pains becomes your uni-
verse. I'm afraid of that. It's hard to get beyond the fact that the body
makes such demands on our attention, and when we're in pain we
forget everything else.

Though I do think suffering can educate a person. Suffering can
take away the armour we have built to sustain our ego, to protect ourselves from others. Suffering makes us helpless. It can make us humble
and permit us to love. It seems scandalous to say suffering is good for
you, but it can be a way of redemption to enable people to love.

Also, the deeper you suffer, the more you can enjoy, it's like mining space inside yourself to be able to hold more. Suffering cultivates an inner depth. The more you cry, the more you can laugh, maybe, because you're finally able to laugh at yourself. And since I've become sick I've been cultivating a rather strange sense of humour. It has to do with a wider perspective on life. It seems that my mental capacities are sharpening, gaining in clarity, while my physical capacities are proportionally degenerating. And for how long is this degeneration going to continue? How long will this last?

The most recent picture a person has of you is the one that sticks. So I'm afraid of being a silly joke of a woman. That's why I really had this question, What am I supposed to give to my children before I die? What am I supposed to leave for them?

My very warmest memory is having tea, well past my bedtime, in my grandmother's kitchen by the coal-burning stove. I was maybe ten or younger. She would look at me, not say anything, just look with very restful eyes. It was a beautiful experience. I remember it perfectly even today. I think this was a big achievement, that my grandmother could look at me with restful eyes, that she wasn't stressed out or thinking about something else or trying to teach me anything or worried about me. We were just sitting in the kitchen over big bowls of tea, and she could just look at me and that was fine. That was enough. It was a kind of doing nothing together. I think that's the kind of time my children want to spend with me now and I want to spend with them, where we're not playing Scrabble or talking about life and death, we're just being together. I don't have to show them anything but love. That's all they need to take away.

The gift I got from my grandmother, when I sat drinking tea with her, is exactly what I would like my children to have. It has nothing to do with my being a model, it's a matter of my receiving them, welcoming them, and silently saying, how wonderful you are. It's simply a look in the eye.

Now, all I need to do is finish my book, which is almost done. I have already taken care of all the practical things. My funeral is paid for. I have arranged for a Mass with lots of singing. After Mass, people will go to an Italian restaurant with good food and lots of wine. Have a party, pull out all the stops! Celebrate my life, enjoy it! I would love that. I think that's how it should end, with a party. Upon one's death I wish that people would remember the life, and it should be a good enough life that it puts a smile on a person's face.

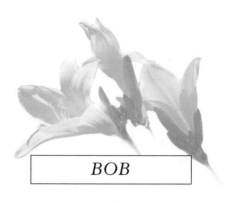

Bob, a thirty-five-year-old man, was dying of AIDS, *and I got his name through a social worker at the* AIDS *Society. He was more than willing to talk. He wanted to hear his own story, to understand his own life. He welcomed the opportunity to be able to relate it to someone who was interested and could put it to some use.*

He lived in the bottom half of a duplex. His house was neat, very precise, with stuffed animals on the bed. The kitchen was spotless. He told me that he washed the kitchen walls every year but that he might not be able to do it this year because of his illness; he didn't think he would have the energy. He was small, about five foot six, compact.

As he was relating his story, he told me about his early abuse by a neighbour. I wanted to push him beyond what he had told me, so I tentatively mentioned, with apologies, that I had read an article about people who had been abused sexually and who, later in life, got sexually excited from events reminiscent of their abuse. He carefully thought about that and then said, "I always wondered why I was attracted to strong men who could harm me. Though they never did."

I had started the interviews at his house, but the last interview was done in the hospital, where he was dressed in new pyjamas and a matching housecoat. He was still uncertain about some details pertaining to the end of his life, and he was still fighting with himself on some issues, but he was content. Ready to go. I felt he was on home

territory. He had worked in a hospital most of his life. Now, he was
finishing his life in a hospital as a patient.

Before, I was a very independent person. I lived alone. I relied on
nobody, was emotionally self-sufficient. My friendships were superficial relationships, dinners once a week with six to eight people. We
never discussed anything profound. Never opened up to each other.

Three years ago, I discovered I wasn't as independent as I thought
I was. After the diagnosis, I had a need to talk about it, and within
the first couple of days I told two friends. But they hardly reacted. It
was like, Oh, you got it, now let's change the subject. They didn't ask
any questions.

It's a very intimate thing, and when your friends don't want to
talk about it, you really feel alone. In the beginning it's more
psychological than physical. Suddenly, I needed people a lot more
than they needed me.

I had been sick for two months with various problems and had
landed in emergency twice. The second time the doctor in the emergency room asked me to have the test. I said, "No."

He came back four or five times to try to convince me to agree
and I wouldn't. The last time, just to get him off my back, I said,
"Okay, do it, but it's going to be negative."

When they drew the blood I started thinking, Maybe it's going to
be positive.

It took a month for me to get the results. That month was hell.
Nothing but the results were of any importance. One day I thought
it was going to be negative, the next day I was convinced it would be
positive. The day the doctor told me, I became numb and just stared
out the window. The first thing I thought of was, Oh, my God, here
I am forty-two years old, and I'm going to die before my dog. The
next thing I thought of was, How am I going to tell my parents? I sat
in a trance for five minutes. The doctor kept talking and I had no
idea what he was saying.

I came home and told my dog. Then I went to bed and stayed

there for a few days. I had to wait several weeks before I could see a specialist, and during that time I started thinking about suicide. The diagnosis meant the end of my world. All I could think of was that I'm going to die. For the first time, work meant nothing to me. Nothing mattered.

After seeing the specialist, I was due to go into hospital for a biopsy. I went shopping for new bathrobes, new pyjamas, everything I would need in the hospital. I packed a suitcase, ready to go, as if I was going on a trip. The biopsy turned out to be just one day. And that packed suitcase has remained untouched in the closet for three years, until now.

Before the biopsy, I felt I had two choices, suicide or fight. I decided to fight this disease right to the end and began to write a diary. I thought, I'm going to be completely forgotten the minute I die. If I can leave the diary to someone, then at least I will have left a trace.

With time the diary has become very important. But I've had problems with it. For close to three years I was just writing down facts, what happened at my doctor's appointment, where I went, what I bought. I haven't put anything more important into the diary because I don't know who's going to read it after I'm gone. My family doesn't know it exists. All my life I've been hiding everything from them and I want that to continue. But something has changed in the past few months. I'm writing more about feelings, about thoughts going through my head. Also, I'm writing every day. Before it was just in spurts. Though I still don't know what I'm going to do with the diary.

I didn't want to tell my parents I was HIV positive because they'd immediately think I was gay. Three months after I got the results, I decided I had to tell them. I got up one Saturday morning and said, "This is the day they're going to find out."

I kept picking up the phone and dialling and dialling. I couldn't dial the last number. I was shaking and crying. I just couldn't do it.

The next day, at eleven-thirty in the morning, I phoned one of my brothers, who lives next door to my parents in the Gaspé, and told him I had AIDS. There was complete silence. I finally said, "Are you still there?"

He said, "Yeah. That's pretty devastating news."

"You should be on this end of the line!" Then I asked, "Would you tell our parents?"

He said, "I'm going right over there to speak to them."

I waited and waited by the phone. Hours passed. I was sure I was never going to hear from them again. To me that call meant acceptance or rejection. It was four o'clock in the afternoon before my phone finally rang.

It was my mother. "How are you? How are things?" She said nothing, as if she didn't know anything.

Finally I said, "Did Russ come over and tell you the news?"

She said, "Yeah, I'm awfully, awfully sorry." Then she said, "That's what we suspected all along."

That shocked me. I thought I had hidden everything so well. Then she asked about different friends, if they were okay. She must have thought I was sleeping with them. Finally she asked if I needed money. And that was it. I would have liked more.

A month later, my mother and father came up for a visit and stayed with me. AIDS was never mentioned. They didn't want to talk about it. The couple of times I touched on it they changed the subject. Still, I felt good they were here. That was the first time I didn't want them to leave. Before, by the end of a week-long visit, I was anxious for them to go. This time, I wanted them to stay.

Everything changes when you get to this stage. All your relationships change. There aren't many invitations anymore. My friends tend to look upon me as a problem or a burden. Steve and I have been friends for twenty-four years, and we're like family to each other. He's also gay, though we've never been to bed together. Now that I need him, I feel I can't count on him. I know he's having a hard time with this. He's going to a support group for friends and relatives of AIDS patients. But I'm having a hard time, too.

I expected a lot from this guy. Steve is like a father substitute for me, though he's only four years older. I can say things to him I wouldn't say to other people. I can really get angry and know he won't walk away. I can also express anger with my father because I know he won't reject me. He and I argued all our lives. I could really scream and yell at him. I did that a lot when I was a teenager. I can also do that with Steve, he's the same way.

I used to be strong, in control of my emotions and always cool. Now I'm completely the opposite. I feel vulnerable, defenceless, and weak all the time. I feel like a little kid, and it's not a good feeling. The more I have to rely on people, the closer I feel to death.

Also, I'm losing my sense of humour. Six months ago, I went in to work for a visit and the first thing they said was, "We really miss your laughter and jokes."

The sense of humour was a big part of me. Humour made people more accepting of me, it gave me a sense of belonging. Humour made me feel comfortable with people and often I didn't feel that comfortable. Also, it helped me have a good relationship with patients. But these days work is the farthest thing from my mind.

Last fall I went through four months of manic activity. Every day I quickly did the housework, took the Metro downtown, and spent much of the day frantically Christmas shopping. I started doing Christmas baskets for all my friends in September and was busy with it right through till Christmas. I was constantly on the run. Steve even said to me, "Why don't you slow down, you're going to exhaust yourself."

I didn't want to think about anything. I felt death was close, and the frantic activity was a way of delaying it. I knew this was going to be my last Christmas and was determined to make it perfect, the best I ever had. I was really looking forward to it. But at the end of Christmas Day, when I went home from Steve's house, I thought, What do I do now? What is there to look forward to?

After Christmas I began chemotherapy. And I fell into a real bout of depression and was so ashamed. I isolated myself from everybody and stayed home except for my twice-a-week visits to the hospital. I didn't want anyone to know how I felt. I sat at home crying for days and days. When someone called, I said, "I'm fine," and tried to sound really up. But I wasn't. As soon as I got off the phone, I was back to crying. I thought if I told someone I was depressed he'd say, "Snap out of it. What are you doing feeling sorry for yourself?"

Yet I felt Steve should have known even if I didn't tell him. And he was rarely even calling. A week could go by without my hearing from him. Much of the winter I was alone.

One day, as the winter was ending, I went to see my doctor and finally told him about being so depressed. He said, "You have the right to be depressed. You've been going through a lot for the past couple of years and you've had no help from anyone. I don't know where you found the strength to deal with all this."

I needed to hear that. It made a big difference because from then on I didn't feel ashamed about it anymore. I realized, Yes, I do have the right to be depressed. But since then I've hardly been depressed because when I'm down I immediately get on the phone and call someone. I'm just sorry I didn't realize earlier that depression was not something to be ashamed of.

Then I started seeing the social worker every week for counselling at the hospital. She said, "You need help and support," and offered to set me up with a buddy. I wasn't very open to this at first and even got upset. A few days later, when Steve called, I flew at him on the phone. I yelled, "You're not around and I need you." Things started changing after that. We started talking more about the whole thing. He even came with me to see the social worker once. I don't think he realized what I was going through.

But I'm still finding him very cold. I guess the friendship has always been like that. He's not the kind of person I could grab and hug. Before, I didn't need him for many things. Now my needs have changed. With Steve one of the big problems is that he'll ask me how I feel about something, and I'll just get started when suddenly he takes over and tells me how he thinks I feel. But I worry about what's going to happen to him when I'm gone. He doesn't make friends easily, he intimidates people. They find him distant. He's from Australia and I'm the only good friend he has. We are like family to each other.

CB

I never felt I belonged in my family. They were totally unaware of my life for the past twenty-eight years. I'm the oldest of four boys, and I've never told my brothers anything. My parents used to ask, "When are you getting married?" In my late twenties I noticed they stopped asking.

When I was living at home, in my teens, my father and I argued about everything. I felt that nothing I did met with his approval. And I wanted it. I knew I was different from my brothers and wanted to fit in. My brothers went fishing. I had no interest in fishing. I liked doing things around the house. I was the reliable, dependable one. I always babysat the younger ones. I was like the little girl in the family and felt my father was disappointed in me. He never verbalized it, but he used to nag, pick. Of course, he did that with all of us.

My father used to drink a lot, and for years I thought it was my fault. He was drunk every time I went home for summer vacations, and I thought it was because I was there. One time I asked my mother, "Is it like this all the time or just when I come home?"

She said, "No, no, it's not because you're home. He's like this all the time."

I hated him for his drinking, probably because I thought I was to blame.

My childhood was horrible. I hated it in the Gaspé, where I grew up, because I was gay. In school you're called "sissy" and "fag." You feel ashamed and try to hide it from everybody. I had no friends. I couldn't get close to anybody because I was afraid they'd find out I was different. I was depressed all the time. I just wanted to get to a city. That's what kept me going.

When I was seventeen, I applied to nursing school from the Gaspé. I never thought of nursing till I saw an ad in the paper. Till then I had no idea what I wanted to do. All I knew was that I wanted to get away from home. Nursing offered me a career, and it was a way out. After I got accepted to nursing school in Montreal, I remember my father saying, "You'll be back in a couple of months."

That made me determined to go through with it so I would never have to come back.

When I got to Montreal, it was scary. I had never been in a city before, I was a typical country bumpkin. I didn't even know you had to wait for the lights to turn green before crossing the street. There were no traffic lights where I came from. During training, I had to live in residence and met a lot of people. Almost all the guys were gay, which was a real shock. Until then I thought I was the only person in the world who was gay. I didn't even know what "gay" meant. At nursing school, I began to understand myself a bit more. We talked about being gay, being attracted to other men. But during those conversations I never admitted I was gay. The others did all the talking. Most of them were comfortable with being gay. A few were as bad as I was. One day a group of us were talking in a guy's room. I was sitting on the bed and another guy sat beside me. He put his arm around me and I got scared. I didn't know what was going on and took off. It was a long time before I openly said I was gay.

When I was eighteen, I got engaged to one of the nursing students. She was from Nova Scotia, and we dated for about a year before I asked her to marry me. But shortly after we were engaged I said to myself, What the hell are you doing? This is wrong. You're going to ruin her life. You're going to ruin your life. If there are any children, what's going to happen to them?

So I called it off. She tried to commit suicide after that. I felt it was my fault. But better that than to go through with the wedding and she'd really know what misery was.

I liked her. Maybe if I hadn't liked her I would have gone through with the marriage. Just to have a facade, a straight front. But I couldn't do it. Later, when I had affairs with married men, I thought back to her and thought, This is how it would have been with me had I gotten married. I'd be sneaking around. She quit her job soon after the suicide attempt and went back to Nova Scotia.

After graduation, I took an apartment and worked at the Douglas Hospital for four years. I spent most of that time on the geriatric unit, except the last six months I switched over to the children's ward to do a permanent night shift. The kids were asleep when I went to work, and they were still asleep when I left in the morning. I needed the night shift to finish my high school credits in the evenings. I had been in such a rush to get away from home that I didn't even finish high school.

Already when I was eight I knew that I was attracted to men. People say you choose, but there's no choice. Who in his right mind would choose to be gay when he could be straight? It complicates your life.

In my teens I developed crushes on other boys. I couldn't do anything or tell anybody about it. I had to keep everything inside. Keeping everything inside carried into my adult life. That's why I never really had a relationship. I had several lovers, but they were just short affairs, nothing lasted. I thought I wanted a relationship, but every time I got into one I felt claustrophobic. I guess I was afraid of the intimacy. I had never had it. All my life if someone just touched my arm I pulled back. I froze, had a panic attack. Unless we were having sex. At work some people were very touchy-feely, and when they talked to me their hands were on my shoulder or arm, and it always bothered me. Though I liked it, I felt I had to pull back, keep a distance. Maybe I thought touching always led to sex.

In my family no one ever touched each other. Even as a kid I don't remember my mother ever putting her arms around me. I never saw my mother and father hug. They argued a lot.

I'm certain I was gay from the minute I was born. Yet I blame a lot of things in my life on having been sexually abused by a neighbour's son when I was five or six years old. He was sixteen at the time. Two years later, his family moved to another town. I don't know how many times the abuse happened. I never told anybody till about two months ago. Even two months ago the only reason I told was because I saw him. I was going into the hospital one day and he was coming out. I immediately recognized him, even though I hadn't seen him in twenty years. I froze. I didn't speak to him and he didn't recognize me. I just stared at him and got very upset. Inside I was a mess.

I had half expected to see him. I'm in touch with Bev, his cousin, who told me he had cancer, plus he's an alcoholic, and he was in Montreal for treatment at the same hospital where I was being treated.

For a long time I felt the sexual abuse had made me gay, but that changed when I was thirty, when I landed in hospital for sixteen days with deep depression. I think the depression was a result of hiding everything. Not being able to accept the fact that I was gay. Plus in my twenties I got into sleeping pills. In the beginning I just took a little Valium to help me sleep because of the night shifts. As time went on, I took more and more Valium. Then I got into bigger things, like Seconal. By the time I hit thirty, I was taking these drugs every day, way above the normal dose. I was on Valium for about eight years. Some days I took as much as seventy milligrams, and a fairly high dose was twenty milligrams a day. I went from doctor to doctor. Never saw the same doctor twice.

In the hospital I was treated with antidepressants, and one day a psychiatrist said to me, "I'm not supposed to give advice, but I'm going to make an exception with you. When you get out of here, go out and enjoy yourself. Enjoy life."

That's all she said, and I listened to her. After that my life changed completely. I got my driver's licence and bought a car. And I started going out to bars.

I didn't tell people about the abuse because I thought they'd just say, Forget it. It happened a long time ago.

That's what I kept telling myself over the years, Forget it. It's over. Put it out of your mind.

I thought everyone else would feel the same way. When I told the social worker two months ago, I was surprised she didn't just brush it off as if it was nothing. She asked questions and dug deeper. It made me feel that I wasn't the only one who thought it was a horrible thing.

I thought a lot about the abuse over the years. From the time it happened, I kept remembering it. I never forgot it. It just kept coming in and out of my head. This was somebody I trusted and looked up to because he was older than me, and he broke the trust. I really hope he dies of cancer. That sounds awful, but I hate him for what he did.

I blame him for my inability to maintain a relationship. I ended all of the relationships except for one. Also, my lovers have always had to be bigger than me. They had to be big, strong, macho men. I had to know they could hurt me. Not that any of them ever did, but I had to know they could. I'm sure this is connected to the abuse. I only became aware of this in the past six months. Now there is no sex, but if the possibility was there, I might go with someone who didn't fit that image.

If he wouldn't have moved away when he was eighteen, the relationship, the abuse, may have continued until I left. I mean, I had no sexual outlet all through my teens. The place was very isolated, there weren't a lot of people around. The majority were elderly. Young people left as soon as they finished school. There was not much work. It was horrible. It was just oral sex. He forced me to perform oral sex on him. He ejaculated in my mouth, and at five or six I didn't know that men ejaculated. It felt so disgusting and dirty. It happened in the woods, and I remember he was holding on to me. He was rough. He didn't hit me, but he was forceful. As soon as it was finished, when he let me go, I ran to a nearby brook. I just kept splashing water in my mouth, trying to clean it out. I was crying and crying. I suppose I felt like a woman feels when she's been raped. You feel so dirty and violated. It was a horrible feeling.

I don't know how long it went on. Maybe two years. This period is all very foggy. If it had continued into my teens, then I suppose it would have meant I wanted it to continue, which would have meant that my anger and hatred toward the whole thing wouldn't be there. When it happened, I had no control over it, I was a little kid. But over the years, when I have thought about it, it was like a turn-on sometimes. I have all sorts of mixed feelings about it.

I always felt I had a certain power over him because of this. I could tell someone and really screw him up. He's a married man with three kids. If I opened my mouth and told the wrong person, this could make a big difference in his life. I never did, but I fantasized. Had I told, it would have meant also revealing a lot about me. That's probably the reason I didn't do it. A couple of months ago, his cousin told me that his twenty-two-year-old son is apparently gay. I suspect the kid may be gay because the father sexually abused him. Though I know that's stupid, if you're gay you're born that way and that's it. I think if I hadn't had that experience of abuse I would still be gay, but I did for many years think that's what made me gay. I never talk about this with my gay friends. But over the years a lot of them had mentioned something about being sexually abused.

I no longer blame him for being gay, for making me gay, but I do blame him for the AIDS. Because I wasn't able to form a relationship with anyone, I was very promiscuous for about eight years. And that's when I caught the AIDS virus. I didn't have sex for sex, it was for the intimacy, the cuddling. With some guys there was more cuddling, and with some guys it was a lot less. And I did get some affection through sex. Usually, after the sex was finished, they'd hold you in their arms, and that was the best part. I think I was having sex just to have a man's arms around me. But that didn't happen all that often. And sometimes I didn't want that either with certain people.

Most of the sex took place in the sauna. There were times I met guys in the bar and we went to the sauna for sex. The sauna was safe. I rarely brought men home. Different guys I knew had been beaten and robbed. Home for me was a haven from everything. I was always glad to get back, to get away from it all. It was safer for me to go to the other guy's house. I figured they wouldn't do much to me in their own home. And as soon as the guy fell asleep, I slipped into my clothes and left. Rarely did I spend the night there. And rarely did I give out my phone number. If they insisted on having it, I changed the last digit. In the past ten years, I have slept with very few guys more than once.

One part of me is very reasonable and responsible, and sometimes I feel like a little child. I'm either one or the other. The adult went to the bar and the child went to the sauna. In the beginning I went to both. There was always the chance you would meet someone in the bar, which usually didn't happen because I would never approach anyone. They had to approach me. And even then I often held back. So that's how this sauna thing started. I realized I could go there and get all the men I wanted, and I didn't have to put on an act. In the sauna, everyone wears a towel, and there is nothing to hide. Everyone is there for the same thing. There are no games. In a bar some people are pursuing and others want to be pursued. After a while I thought, I can't be bothered with these games. Skip that part and let's get right to the sex.

When it came to meetings, I always played a very passive role. I never went after somebody. They had to come after me. They had to do all the work. I was very shy. When I went anywhere I just stayed in a corner quietly and never spoke to anyone unless they spoke to me. Often when I went into a room I would become fixated on a certain man. I'd make eye contact with him. He'd see me watching him. But he had to approach me. A lot of guys have told me they were afraid to approach me because I had an angry look. I wasn't aware of it. They said, "I was afraid to speak to you because I thought you might reject me."

I was a loner. I did almost everything alone. Even went to the bars alone. I just went two nights a week, when I didn't have to work the next day. The first several times I went to a bar, I was terrified. After about ten visits to the same place, I started to feel much more relaxed. I always went to the same place because it was too difficult to start over somewhere else. In gay bars, there are always people coming from out of town. And most gays were not like me, they didn't go to the same bar all the time. So for me the same bar didn't really have a regular crowd.

I did try to have relationships. The longest lasted about two years. He was quite wealthy, from a family with money. He was a big man, six foot six. When I met him he was working with a company in Ontario, and he had a fancy apartment here in Montreal. He was very much in the closet, he didn't want anyone to know. He flew in every second weekend, and I moved in to stay with him on weekends. He took me to fabulous restaurants. Six months into the relationship, he moved out to Vancouver. He paid for my ticket to fly there every second weekend. I was twenty-six at the time, and the whole affair was like an adventure. He was a nice guy, very caring and gentle.

One day I asked him about a ring he always wore on his finger. It was an ugly ring that didn't match the rest of him. He dressed well, was very classy. I said, "Grant, why do you wear that ring?"

"My son gave it to me. He made this ring."

I said, "Your son? I didn't know you had a son."

"I don't. I was married, had a son, and he died."

"Of what?"

"Leukemia."

"How old was he?"

"Eight." Then he said, "And I don't want to talk about it."

I would have liked to talk more about it. I would have liked to know what kind of a relationship he had with his son. Was it a loving relationship or was it like what I had with my father?

Whenever I saw a movie, either on TV or in the theatre, where a father and son were close and they hugged each other, I became very emotional and started crying. I couldn't help it. The tears just flowed. It's always been like that.

Soon after Grant, I met the only person I ever loved. I was in the bar and noticed Terry sitting across the room. I liked what I saw, he was tall and broad-shouldered, and I went for it. He was the only guy I ever approached. We spent the whole night in a corner, and I never shut up. I told him my whole life story in three or four hours. And he listened. He was from New York state and owned a funeral home. We went out for about a year. He was such fun, always so up and perky and on the run. I felt he was the opposite of me. He was exciting. We danced a lot. We laughed a lot. He had a very good sense of humour. He was extremely affectionate. We'd spend hours just lying on the couch, holding each other. It was the best. I loved everything about him. When we broke up, I didn't think I could go on. I was devastated. I suppose it could have continued, but he started going out with other people and I couldn't tolerate that.

I'm glad I've always been attracted to macho men. I never wanted to do it with a boy. I've been terrified of kids all my life. I don't trust myself with them. I think I'm afraid I might do that, or I might get the desire to. My friends know I don't want kids around me. They don't know why. When they come here, they don't bring their children. When I go to see them, it's usually when the kids are at school or out with their father. I want nothing to do with children. And I know that's because of the sexual abuse.

Though for nearly ten years, in my early thirties, I fantasized a lot about having a son. I never told this to anyone, I just kept it inside. I wanted a son because I wanted to raise him the way I was not raised. I wanted to raise him the right way, to give him all the things I never got from my father. Of course, I also wondered if I could tolerate it, if I could trust myself. Would I abuse him the way I had been abused? I considered adoption or having a foster child, but then I thought it would be too complicated being gay and alone. Then I thought maybe a single girlfriend would want to have a child. But I didn't actually do anything about it. In the end I decided it's better that I don't have a son.

In a way my patients were like my children. I took good care of them and grew quite attached to some of them. Some were very special to me. Work was always the number-one priority in my life. No matter what I did outside, nothing interfered with work. I had to be on time. I had to know more than everyone else. Since most of the time I was the only male nurse, I had to be better than the others. Whenever there was a seminar, I had to be there. If the others didn't know something they knew they could always ask me.

Sometimes the work was hard psychologically. When psychiatric and geriatric patients got agitated, they became verbally abusive. I took that personally, and it could be very upsetting, particularly if it was a patient I liked. Though I think being in the hospital among these patients might have felt like home. My father had also been verbally very abusive.

But at least I could have a certain relationship with the patient that I couldn't ever have with my father. The patient was the one person with whom I could express affection. If someone wanted a hug, I gave it to them. Also, since I always wanted to be touched, I sensed when a patient wanted and needed to be touched. Sometimes I rubbed a patient's back while talking to them. I couldn't do that with anyone else. I could pick up patients' needs. And their response was very gratifying. The geriatric patients rarely remembered your name, and yet I was the only person whose name they could ever remember.

There have been several special patients over the years. Five years ago, an eighty-six year old lady called Olive was brought in. She had had surgery and weighed about sixty-five pounds. We didn't think she was going to live. She was quite confused most of the time, but after a while she learned my name and used to call, "Bob, Bob." I was the only staff whose name she knew. She didn't even remember some of her relatives' names when they came in. But she knew mine. After surgery she went through a course of physio, and I was told to walk her every day on the ward. Another nurse and I walked her to the toilet and back to her chair three times a day. Eventually she was steady enough that I could walk her alone. One day her family came in and I was walking her down the hall and they were amazed. They said, "We were told she was never going to walk again." Everyone said she had only begun to walk because of the work I had done with her.

She was my favourite patient. I was getting a lot of affection back from her. She kissed me often. I remember once I had been away on vacation for two weeks. On my first morning back, I went into her room with the breakfast tray, and she cried out, "Bob, you're back!"

I didn't think she would realize I was gone.

She said, "Come here."

I went over.

"Come closer, I want to tell you something."

As soon as I got over to the bed she just reached up, grabbed me by the head, pulled me down, and gave me a big kiss, saying, "Don't ever go away again." I almost cried. She died last July. I was sorry I couldn't go to her funeral.

She reminded me of my paternal grandmother, who lived next door to us. She was very important to me. I was one of her favourite grandchildren. She was always giving me little gifts. I used to like going to her house and staying overnight. They had a big house, and everything was always neat. She had an old wood stove, and when you got up in the morning, there was a big bowl of oatmeal sitting on top of the stove.

My grandfather was similar to my father. There was absolutely nothing between us. Neither was there anything between my father and his mother. I think my father was also starving for affection. This lack of communication is a learned behaviour that's passed down from generation to generation.

My father and grandfather had a carpentry business, a big shop where they made furniture, windows and doors. When I was a kid I'd do odd jobs, like paint window frames, to make a little extra money. They never talked about anything, just work. They tolerated each other, I guess. One of my brothers, Russ, who I called about my diagnosis, inherited the business.

My father built our house himself, and it was never finished. My grandparents' house was all finished, that's what I liked about it. Our house always seemed to be missing things, like a door from this or that room. And our house was small. My three brothers slept in one bedroom upstairs, my parents had the other bedroom, and I had a tiny bedroom downstairs to myself. I was glad I had that, but for years I had no bedroom door. Though my mother was a pretty good housekeeper, we didn't have the nicer things my grandparents had, like attractive furniture with no scratches. In their house everything was in good condition. In our house the furniture was badly abused, I guess because there were four boys. My grandparents had a dining room and we didn't. We always ate in the kitchen. I suppose all that wouldn't have bothered me if there had been some love and affection in our house. I always felt something was missing, and I thought it was the nicer things, like the good furniture, the doors on the rooms.

My grandmother was the only person with whom I was comfortable. With her there were things that just didn't need to be said. Neither of us had to say, "I love you." I felt her love when I was with her. After I left the Gaspé, we wrote to each other once a week. Though I never told her I was gay.

I was about twenty-five when she died, and her death was very rough on me. I cried a lot at her funeral. That was the one time I lost control. I missed her for a long time. It's probably because of my grandmother that I liked working with geriatric patients. I seemed to get on well with them, a lot better than with the younger ones. And

I got along much better with the female patients than the male patients. I hated having male patients. Yet with some I did have a good relationship. But the relationships with male patients took a long time to develop, and I was always very surprised to find out that a particular male patient liked me.

I still remember one patient from the time I was twenty-three. He was about forty and had cancer in his spine and lungs. By the time he arrived on my ward, one arm had been amputated. Every night he watched *The Tonight Show* till twelve-thirty, and then I had to go to his room to position him for the night. If I didn't go, he would ring for me. Because of the cancer in his spine, you had to be very, very careful when you moved him. There had to be certain pillows in certain spots behind him and in between his legs. It took six pillows to get him in position. After I had done it a couple of times, he said to me, "You do it so much better than anyone else."

The two nights I was off every week there were always problems. He couldn't get comfortable. He used to say, "When you're not here, I can't sleep. The others can't fix me up the way you do."

He had been there for three weeks when, one night, soon after I came into work on my night shift, he started hemorrhaging from his lungs. We immediately began working on him. There was blood everywhere. The room was a mess. Half of us were covered in blood. The man was terrified. And blood was squirting out all over the place. He opened his mouth and the blood shot to the foot of the bed. I never saw so much blood. There was blood on the walls of the room. It was horrible. And he was frantic. He wanted us to do all we could, to do more than we could. And there was nothing we could do. He was dead in half an hour. This took everything out of me for a while. And I had gotten to know him and liked him, which made it worse. That night has stayed with me all these years.

When I first started working in geriatrics, we were averaging about fifty deaths a year. Sometimes, as the patient was dying, I sat beside them holding their hand. And often I didn't even notice they had died. It was so peaceful. At one point I'd look up to see he or she was gone. And then I didn't leave immediately. I remained with the person a while longer.

Death is an intimate thing. It's important to have the right person with you when you're dying. I've thought a lot about this lately. I don't want to be alone when my time comes. For some reason I don't want my family there. I want John to be there.

John was assigned to me as a buddy six or seven weeks ago. The social worker put the two of us together. He reminds me very much of Terry, the way he moves, the way he walks, the way he does things. I may be in love with him. I'm beginning to think it's possible to love someone without the sex. John and I discuss our emotions, and I've never done that with anyone before. Terry and I didn't discuss emotions, but I did tell Terry I loved him. He was the only person I said that to. Now I constantly tell John that he's special and I like him. I've never been able to say that to people. This illness has given me the opportunity to be intimate, to express my feelings.

With John I can cry, and I would never have cried in front of my friends. I can go to John and say, I need a hug. I would be afraid to ask a friend for a hug. You fear rejection. Of course, I don't know what I would have done if one of my friends had come to me asking for a hug. I couldn't imagine giving Steve a hug. I seem to have had a knack for finding people who are a lot like me, distant, definitely not touchy-feely.

Now I know who I want to have the diary. Steve knows about it, but the day I told him he said, "I don't want it. Don't leave it to me."

I am leaving the diary to John after I die. He is a writer, so maybe he can use it for something. I don't care what he does with it as long as he keeps it.

Everything changes with AIDS. Before, work was my priority, now it's the last thing I want to do. Before, the more responsibility I had on the ward, the better I liked it. After the results, I didn't want any responsibility, and half the time I didn't even want to be there. Even my relationship to the dog has changed. I pay less attention to her lately. She comes around and wants to sit on my knee and I don't want her. She has been so important to me, especially through this.

When I first got her, this dog was very frustrating, she wouldn't come near me. I showered her with affection, and she wanted no part of me for the first month. If she was on the couch and I sat down, she left. She was throwing up all over the house. The minute I turned my back, there were puddles everywhere. I thought, I can't seem to bond with this dog, what's wrong here?

Then I decided, I can't go on with this and took her back. The dog spent one night at the clinic, and I felt so guilty I had to go back and get her. After that there were no more problems. She suddenly changed. That first month, I think she was testing me to see how far she could go. She did everything wrong. Like a kid. When I brought her back home again, I think she realized, It doesn't matter what I do, he still wants me, he still loves me.

Getting Lady meant having something to love, to be close to. Her name is supposed to be Lady but I call her Baby. It's probably the most solid relationship I ever had. Except for one night, we haven't been apart for eight years. I once ended an affair because the guy didn't like the dog. One of my biggest fears was what will happen to her once I'm gone? I've asked my parents to take her for whatever life she has left. With my parents, she'll be looked after, she'll be well fed, probably overfed. We always had a dog, and the dog was well treated. In some ways the dogs were better treated than I was.

There are a few things I regret in my life. One is not getting any affection from my parents, another is that I will not be able to retire. I would have liked to travel some more. I did travel, and I loved it. I've been to Florida, Hawaii, Jamaica. I won a trip for two to Japan in 1970 for eight days, to the World's Fair. First class all the way, with everything paid for. I asked my father to come with me because he had been a prisoner of war in Japan during World War II. But he said he absolutely didn't ever want to go back. So I took my mother instead. We had a good time. And for a while we were closer.

Whenever I travelled, it was always first class. And I always bought new clothes before I went on a trip. I said, "I live like a peasant all the time, when I go away I have to stay at the Hilton."

I have champagne taste but can only afford beer. My whole life I always lived from paycheque to paycheque. I worked very hard for what little I had, and when I went on a trip I had to do it right.

❧

To a certain extent the past sixteen months have been like retirement. I enjoy not having to get up in the mornings. I can do whatever I want, whenever I want. When I first stopped working, I really missed it for a couple of months, then something changed. One day my doctor was filling out the insurance papers and came to a section where they ask when you expect to return to work. He asked me what to put. I said, "I don't think I'm ever going back."

And he said, "You're right, you're never going back."

These past sixteen months have given me the opportunity to be with myself, to get to know myself. I've had time to think. Though I'm not sure it's all that good. You pick up things you'd rather not, it's painful. I'm not sure I want to know who I am. There seem to be so many things I can't figure out. I'm a mystery to myself.

This illness has taken over my life completely, I'd be afraid to give it up now. If they found a cure for AIDS tomorrow, I don't think I would take it. Isn't that weird? It's a full-time job staying alive. You spend your whole day planning what you're going to eat, and you've got to take ten pills at this time, twelve pills at that time, and you've got your doctor's appointments. All my time is spent taking care of myself. I've never done that before, and it's a lot harder than I thought it would be.

I'm getting more from this AIDS than I bargained for. Until I joined the support group, I thought I was the only person going through all these things. Now I know they're all going through a depression at times, they're all going through pain and they all feel like giving up sometimes. It makes a big difference knowing you're not alone.

I was afraid to go to the group the first time. I expected to see people looking really bad, with things on their faces. I thought, this could be a real downer, and I was depressed enough. After an hour, I said, "I belong to this group."

For a long time, I really didn't feel I belonged anywhere. I have never shared anything with anybody till I started meeting with the social worker and going to the group. I kept everything inside. So

I've never had anyone say, "I know what you mean, I've been through that." You need permission to feel these things.

I've accepted the disease now, it's a part of me. That's why if they would find a cure I wouldn't take it. I've changed so much since I was diagnosed HIV positive, and I like the change. Now if I say good-bye to a man, I hug and kiss him on the street. I would never have allowed that to happen before. Now I don't care who sees or what they think, and I like that. The disease has allowed me to be myself.

I feel the time I have left now is my time. I don't want to do things that I don't want to do anymore. If I'm somewhere and I'm not having a good time, I won't stay and just tolerate it. I'm leaving, and I don't care what anyone thinks. This time is precious to me. I can't waste it doing things I don't want to do. Before, I tolerated anything no matter how miserable I was. That's what people expect you to do. And I expected myself to do the right thing.

I've decided to tell you something, something I would never have thought of telling anybody, something that I've always been ashamed of. I'm afraid people will judge me for it, though I know I judge myself first. And I'm probably much more critical of myself than anyone else would be.

I want to tell you how many men I've been to bed with. In excess of three thousand. Though I only went out a couple of times a week, I averaged more than one a night. I didn't get everything I wanted from the first one, so I had to keep trying with others until I got what I wanted, which was affection. So many couldn't give it. Lately I feel less ashamed of the promiscuity. I'm no longer ashamed of my need for affection.

The abuse made me feel dirty, disgusting. I've never been able to express the anger I've felt about it, and I think I turned it against myself. The promiscuity was part of it. I had very low self-esteem, and when you're promiscuous, you're letting people use your body. Though I also wanted something from them, I still felt that I was the one being used.

Emotional pain is much worse than physical pain. When there's physical pain, at least you know you're alive. But sometimes I think, maybe the pain is all in my head. For a while some of the nurses in the hospital convinced me that my breathing problem was caused by fear and depression. I was sure I was bringing this on myself. Then a month ago, Marie, my favourite nurse, said, "Your breathing is really bad."

I said, "It's like this all the time."

She said, "Are you sure it's not anxiety?"

I felt really disappointed that of all people she would say that. Marie is my favourite nurse. I don't get along well with the other nurses. Once she said to me, "There's only one like you." She makes me feel important.

After I had seen the doctor, I made a point of telling her that I will have to go back on chemotherapy because of the lung deterioration. I explained that my breathing problem wasn't anxiety. I felt a little angry at having to justify it. But I wouldn't confront Marie about anything because I'm afraid she might reject me.

I think I get too attached to these people, to my doctor as well. I know that if it weren't for Jason, my doctor, I wouldn't be alive today. Yet I can confront him but not Marie. I know that, no matter what I say to him, he can't drop me as a patient, he's not going to reject me. I got really upset near the end of February. Marie phoned to say my appointment for my chemo had to be changed because Jason was going away for a month. Just a month earlier he had said, "You have to give up all responsibility for your health because that's my responsibility now."

Then he goes away for a month. Immediately I thought, I'll never survive the month without him. The breathing got even worse. I had to go into hospital, and they put me through all sorts of tests. They thought I had pneumonia again. But it was just a panic attack.

For the past six months I've realized I'm going to die. Before it was easy to say to people, "I'm dying," because I didn't really believe it. Now I do. Before, when I'd get into an argument with Steve, I'd say, "You don't understand, I'm dying, that's what's wrong."

I stopped saying that. Probably because now I really believe it. It sunk in. I remember going through a period of denial, a period of anger. Of course, I kept it all inside. I wanted to kill someone, I was so angry. In the beginning, I blamed the doctor who had talked me into having the AIDS test. I hated this man for a long time. I remember he kept coming back to me in emergency, trying to convince me to have that test. For a long time, every time I felt anger his face came into my mind. Then I started thinking, Who could I have gotten this from? I wanted someone to blame. Then I realized that, after having had all these men, there was no way of knowing who I got it from.

Then I wondered how many years I've had it and who I gave it to. Maybe I've given it to many people. I had the phone number of one person I had been together with fairly recently. I called him. When I told him, he was a little surprised, but he thanked me for telling him. He's an Anglican priest. I met him in the sauna. The affair went on for about a year and a half, occasional get-togethers. He has a church, and I've been to his house.

He didn't tell me he was a priest in the beginning. First he told me he was a social worker. After a couple of times, he told me everything, including the whole story about the wife and the daughter. He was afraid someone would find out about him. He said it would ruin his career. I knew what he was going through because I've also hidden everything most of my life. But he's terrified that he has the virus, and he won't go to be tested. Last year his wife left him and took their daughter. Now he's alone. Since I've told him that I'm HIV positive, he hasn't had sex with anyone. He calls me once a month, and we'll have a long conversation.

Last February he called and asked me over to his house. We spent the evening together before the fireplace. He held me in his arms. It was nice. When I think about it, I have had a lot more support than I realize. Friends have been a lot better than I should have expected.

Steve phoned me last night, and we were on the phone for two hours. We had a good talk about a lot of things, which is unusual. We talked about when I will die. He said, "I'm really going to miss you when you're gone." It's the first time he's ever said that.

I spent last Christmas Day at his house. There were six of us and it was the perfect Christmas, just as I wanted it. I told this to Steve, and I said, "But there was just one thing missing."

He said, "What?"

"We've always spent Christmas Day together, and every year, when you open the gift I give you, you run across the room, throw your arms around me, and kiss me on the cheek. This past Christmas you didn't do that, and I was really expecting it. Before, I always felt uncomfortable when you did that, and I never hugged you back, I never put my arms around you. This year I was going to hug you back when you came over to kiss me. And you didn't do it. Why?"

He said, "I don't know."

After Christmas, last February, my parents came for a visit, and all the time they were here I kept thinking of only one thing. I wanted to ask my father for a hug. Every evening, as they were leaving to return to their hotel, I was planning to say to my father, "Give me a hug, you old devil." Something like that. I wanted this hug to the point that I was trembling, shaking. And I couldn't ask for it. I really tried so hard, but I just couldn't get the words out. I think I was afraid he would say no.

I don't ever remember touching my father in my whole life. Never even shook hands. I can probably count on one hand the number of times my mother has kissed me. And most of that was when they were here in February. Then she kissed me every day that she saw me. It felt good.

But I really wanted that hug from my father. I think that hug would have meant acceptance of who I am and what I am, the way I am. It would have meant approval. It would have meant everything. It's weird. A lot of my life I thought I hated my father, but I'm finding out it's the other way around. I'd like to tell him that I love him, and I'd like to tell my mother that, too, and I never have. I'm going to write them a letter, I've been planning to do this for a while. They will get it after I die. It's the best I can do. I'm afraid to simply ask for that hug while I'm still alive. I don't know why, maybe I'm ashamed of needing that hug so much.

Sometimes, when I went home to the Gaspé for holidays, I felt like an intruder. The only thing I had to look forward to was knowing that my father and I would sing and play old country songs together. The music gave me a sense of belonging while we were doing it. Even though a lot of the time we were playing he was drunk or drinking. But it didn't matter whether he was drunk or sober, at least we were together.

We didn't just play at home. Sometimes we performed at other people's houses. Also, we were often asked to perform at the town hall for the Christmas concert. Sometimes I gave a concert alone. People always told me I played well. My father never told me, yet I always knew he was proud of me for that. Often when people came to the house he pushed me to play for them.

I started playing the piano at my grandparents' house when I was quite young. My grandmother paid for piano lessons. And I played for her. She really enjoyed it. She was very proud of my playing. Everybody was very encouraging, especially my father. I think that's why I continued to play.

One day, when I was twelve, my father came home and announced that he knew someone who had an old piano for sale, for $100. He said, "I was wondering if you might want it."

I had $100 in the bank, just. And I bought the piano myself. After that, he played the guitar beside me while I played the piano. We did this almost every day. That's the only thing we ever did together. When he wanted to play, he went into the room where the piano was and started tuning the guitar. Then I knew it was time to join him. There was nothing said. When we played together, it was peaceful because we weren't fighting and were as intimate as we ever could be. Sometimes, when we sang, he stood behind me with his hand on my shoulder. It was the only thing, the only time that I had with him, the only way I could get his attention. I had the music over my brothers, they didn't do any of this.

Over the years, my father has often said he wished he had a daughter. He has four sons and he's not close to any of us. He feels that if he would have had a daughter he would have had a relationship with her, like a father-daughter relationship. He's aware that there is nothing between him and us, I know that. I think it must make him feel really alone, maybe unwanted even. I guess he feels a lot like I do.

About six years ago my father sold his guitar. While working with the electric saw, he cut the ends of two of his fingers on his right hand. So for the past six years, when I went back home, he couldn't play the guitar. I played the piano for both of us. He never actually asked me to play. At some point I went into the room and started playing. Then he came in to join me. Or he went in and started puttering around, playing a few notes. It was so pathetic because he couldn't really play the piano. So I went in and said, "Move over, move over." Then he either stood around or pulled up another chair while I played.

If my parents would have been more open and affectionate, it would have changed a lot of things for me. For one, the promiscuity might never have happened. But then even the promiscuity I look back on as something positive because it was the closest thing to affection I ever got. I wasn't affectionate to others, either, because that's the way I was raised. I wanted it yet couldn't give it. Now I can. Knowing that I'm dying has given me a lot of courage.

I'm enjoying life more than I ever did. I'm surprised each morning that I'm still here. Even if it's a bad day I'm glad to be here. There's an urgency about everything. Each day is precious, even a day I'm depressed. Before, if something would have gone wrong, I would have just given up. I didn't give a damn whether I lived or died. I don't think I was really living all those years. I just started living lately. And I feel there are certain things I still need to do and know before the end.

There's got to be a right way to die, but I don't know what that is yet. You have to do it right the first time, you don't get a second chance. I'm working on that. I'm refining the right way to die as I get closer. I always have to be organized. Before I go on a trip, everything has to be prepared and ready. That's how I want to die, organized and ready. I want to have about a week where I know I'm dying. There will be certain people I will want to see because I will have something to tell them. I don't know what yet. And I want to say goodbye to everyone, including my parents. During that week, I will not want to spend time by myself. I want people with me all the time. By then I will have done enough thinking. And at the last minute I want the right person to be there, not a stranger.

If I would see the guy who molested me, I would like to tell him that I hate him, that he had no right to do what he did to me. Lately, I don't hate him as much as I did even six months ago. Had I met him six months ago, I would have wanted to kill him. Now, I don't know.

I'm beginning to feel a sense of completion about my life, like the cycle is coming to an end. The circle is about to close. I feel physically weak, and I don't feel very good about my body now. But what I'm losing physically I'm gaining mentally.

I spoke to John yesterday and told him this could be it. I've been in hospital for fourteen days now and have had fever every day. First I had pneumonia in the left lung, and now I have pneumonia in the right lung as well. And I really have problems breathing. Steve certainly thinks I'm dying because every time he leaves he gives me a hug, and he never does that except on Christmas Day. My parents called to say they were coming down to spend a week.

If this is it, I'm ready. Death is going to be a good long rest.

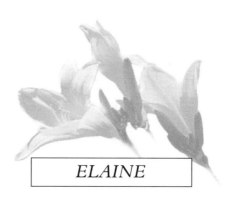

ELAINE

I got Elaine's name from a hospital social worker. Elaine, forty-six, was part of a cancer support group, and she often came as a volunteer to the oncology ward.

When I called her, she enthusiastically agreed to participate. She wanted to do the interviews at my house, since it was close to the hospital where she regularly had to go to see her doctor or her group or other patients. She showed up in a sweatsuit, explaining that the cancer drugs had been ballooning her for months. She said she felt like the Michelin man or Mr. Clean. She was about five foot three or five foot four. Dressing well had once been a source of pride, but she had to let that go because chemotherapy and other drugs were constantly changing her body.

She was always in a good mood and told her story with a sense of perspective and humour. It was obvious that she had come to terms with her various dilemmas, her cancer. Once-painful situations were now viewed from a distance. She laughed at herself when she talked about a doctor she had a crush on. Though she realized this was clearly not going to blossom into a romance, she had hopes that something might happen. Here she was, walking the tightrope of death, still dreaming dreams, yet whether these dreams came true or not made no difference to her anymore.

Elaine was certainly willing to die, but she wanted to use all the weapons at her disposal to fight the cancer, and she wanted the doctors to give her new, untried treatments. She offered herself up to the medical profession as a guinea pig in the hope that their research would find new drugs to fight this disease.

When I was fifteen, I had my life planned out till the age of ninety-four. I was going to get married, live in a house with a white picket fence, and have two children, a boy and a girl. The father has the son and the mother has the daughter. I didn't want three children because I would have worried that two would be close and one would be left out. The family of four fits. My husband and I were going to grow old together, side by side in rocking chairs. My life was going to be uneventful, simple, ordinary. And I did have what I wanted for a long time.

Now, I go day by day. Maybe I'll plan for next week, but I try not to. Sometimes I'm afraid of having too much hope, I worry that I'm not protecting myself. Most of the time I know I'm dying, so if you know you're dying you're protected. But sometimes I say to myself, I feel like a normal person. Maybe I'm not dying. And I get scared. When other people talk about next year, next month, or the next holidays, I stop talking because I don't have the right to that conversation. And people always talk future. Do you know how many people have talked to me about grandchildren since my daughter announced her engagement? They don't know the pain they are causing me. I don't say, "I'm not going to be alive for the grandchildren," because that's going to make them feel bad, so I just sit there and smile. But when I'm not protecting myself then I allow myself to think about the grandchildren, and I think, Who knows?

For a long time I didn't have a lot, but it was exactly the way I had planned it. The little perfect family of four, the ballet lessons, the hockey lessons. Then, five years ago I was diagnosed with breast cancer, stage one, minimal cancer, nothing to worry about.

I was hysterical. Cancer was not a word in my vocabulary. All I knew was that cancer kills people. And breast cancer means you lose your breast. I didn't want to be deformed. I didn't want anything to happen, I just wanted things to be the way they were. At the time, there couldn't be anything worse for me than breast cancer. There was worse.

When I checked into the hospital, three weeks after the diagnosis, I was quite in control. One of the residents called me a model patient. I did what I had to do. I told the staff what I wanted. I put makeup on every morning and wore nice robes. But my husband showed no warmth, no caring. Ten years earlier, when I had a hysterectomy, Peter was the perfect husband. Eighteen hours a day by my bed, wet washcloths on my forehead. This time he sat with his back to me. He didn't even wish me good luck before the operation.

After the operation, the cancer didn't look invasive. They didn't do the lymph nodes. The biopsy results indicated the cancer had only slightly invaded. Five days later, they took me back into surgery to do the lymph nodes. This time, the breast was a little deformed, but that was okay.

My doctor and I had meetings about possible treatments, and I realized no one knew what the right treatment was. I had a list of twenty questions, and nineteen of them he answered, "We really don't know."

I said to myself, My daughter could be sitting at this desk one day, and I'd like them to know. So I chose to participate in an experimental study. I was given radiation and an unidentified pill. The Friday before I was to start radiation, my husband announced he was leaving me. I was forty-three.

When Peter left, it felt like it was the end of my life. I felt robbed. Not only did I lose him, but I lost one of the most important things in my life, the family unit.

I had twenty good married years before he went through a typical midlife crisis. He was very conservative, undershirt twelve months a year, the shirt buttoned to the neck. He took a shower at eleven, at ten after eleven had a snack, and by eleven-fifteen he was in bed. Then he became financially successful, and one day he came home with his shirt open to his waist. I couldn't believe my eyes. He became loud. Before, I was the loud one. His schedule became erratic. He came home late. Went to bed late.

When we were young, a lot of what attracted him to me was my strength, my ability to do certain things that he felt he couldn't do. As he gained confidence, which came with success, he resented my strength. I didn't change, I offered exactly what I had always offered. Had he been a more communicative person, he might have said, "I no longer want that from you." And you adjust your relationship. But I didn't know he no longer wanted it. He became very distant, cool, and even stopped talking to me for a few months.

A little after these changes began, I had my son's bar mitzvah and my daughter's sweet sixteen. I said to myself, "I'm going to have to deal with this later."

After the two events, I got the kids ready for camp. When they left, we went to a friend's house, and Peter excused himself after supper and left.

My friend asked, "What's with him? Where did he run off to?"

"I think he's seeing someone."

"You're out of your mind. This is the last man in the world who would ever do this." She was shocked. "Who?"

"It has to be someone who would have gone after him because he doesn't have the courage to run after someone. There's really only one person I can think of, this girl in the office."

We looked up her address in the phone book and drove to her house. There was his car. I opened the car door and vomited on the street. I can't begin to describe the nausea I felt.

For a week I thought about what happened and then wrote him a letter saying, either we go for help or he moves out. He was not ready to make a move, so he agreed to go for help. We went to a psychiatrist, and Peter complained that I write on my Kleenex box. I remember the psychiatrist saying, "After twenty-two years of marriage, is that the only thing you can tell me that your wife does wrong?"

But really, when you decide not to love someone, you simply don't love them. It doesn't matter if I did anything right or wrong, he didn't want me.

A few months into the treatment, the psychiatrist had a nervous breakdown, and he wasn't available for a year. No one told us he was going to be off for so long, and we kept waiting and waiting. During this time, my father was getting sicker and sicker. So this bullshit was set aside and we were at a truce.

My husband was very close to my father. Peter had in my parents what he never had in his. They worked together for sixteen years before my father began to have heart problems and retired. My mother brought them lunch every day, and every day they sat down to eat together.

When we got married, my father said to Peter, "I have nothing to offer you right now, but if I have, you'll have." I was nineteen and Peter was twenty-one when we got married. He was honest and decent, and those were qualities I was attracted to. Also, he was very cute, and when you're young, cute is important. We were in love and times were good. A family business, dealing in import office equipment, was started out of my parents' basement. We worked days, nights, weekends together to build it up. And Peter and I did everything else together, paint the fence, the walls, put up the wallpaper. We were a team. We were buddies. When I had my daughter, I stopped doing the business nights and weekends, but I did the accounts receivable at home when she was sleeping, which was a little lonely because I wasn't with him anymore. When I gave birth to my son, I stopped altogether. By then my sister and brother-in-law had also joined the business.

A year after things started to go crazy with Peter, after he began his philandering, my father was close to death. Before he died, the whole thought of death and dying had been terrifying for me. I always thought death was an action verb, like, you *die*. But what my father did was stop living. He didn't do anything, he just slowly stopped breathing. I arrived at the hospital with my mother at seven-thirty AM and he died at twelve-thirty PM. I cried from seven-thirty to twelve-thirty non-stop. When he died, suddenly I became calm. My sister and mother were hysterical. I was silent. There was nothing else to cry about. It was over. While I was trying to keep him from dying, I was in a panic that it might slip out of my control. Once he was dead, there was nothing else for me to do. And the body that was there wasn't my father anymore. It seemed like he had left his body. My mother and sister were shrieking. I didn't let out a peep, not a tear.

I held my mother, and Peter came over and held the two us. There were times when he was caring. I sometimes think of the last five years of our marriage as having been awful, but there were times when he went back to being normal. For a while after my father's death, he was good to me.

When my father was buried, I didn't feel it was my father going underground. Even now when I go to the cemetery, I don't really feel much. I feel more when I'm driving in my car and we have a little chat. His dying made me unafraid to die. I used to say I could never go in the ground. Now, hey, I'm not going to be there, do what you have to do.

One afternoon, two or three years after my father's death, after I had already been diagnosed with breast cancer, I called Peter to ask what time he was coming home for supper.

"I'm coming home but not for supper," he said. "We have to talk."

By the time he came home, I was a basket case. He told me he was leaving, moving out.

"I can't do this alone," I cried. "How can you leave?"

I was terrified of being left alone. I was pleading, begging him to stay. Then he said, "There is someone else."

That was like a barrel of ice-cold water over my head. He was finally admitting he had betrayed me. Before he had sworn there was no one else, and I had hoped for that one percent chance. Now I knew it was over. The tears and hysteria stopped. I simply said, "Take your things and get out of my house."

After he left, I got progressively worse. My kids were left to deal with a mother who has cancer and a father who is a liar and a sneak. I fell into a state of clinical depression. The only reason I didn't go into a total depression was because I had to go for radiotherapy every day.

CB

Before I got sick, I was very active in our synagogue. Was on the Soviet Jewry committee. I sat on the school committee. I was a Jewish Education counsellor. I was in community theatre. I was the president of the rifle club. You name it and I've done it. Innocent, normal things. After Peter left, I resigned from all my activities and went to a psychologist once a week for a year and a half.

Then I had to rebuild my life. I joined the cancer support group in the hospital and did volunteer work on the oncology unit. Being a volunteer was an opportunity to educate myself about this disease. I went to lectures on cancer, and working with patients, listening to them, made me very knowledgeable.

A few months after I began work as a volunteer, my doctor went to Ethiopia for a year and gave me to a colleague. He said it was only going to be for three checkups and then he will be back. Nothing to worry about. Soon after he left, I began to feel quite sick. A week before my next checkup, my daughter was graduating from McGill and my son was graduating from Vanier. I was so happy, yet I was so worried. I went to my checkup with a list of complaints. The doctor said everything was fine. I was not convinced.

One night I was driving downtown listening to a medical program on the radio. It was an interview with a liver specialist who was describing the symptoms for liver metastasis. I realized that's exactly what I had. I drove straight to the hospital, went upstairs to the cancer unit, pressed this doctor I had heard about against the wall and said, "I think my cancer has metastasized to my liver, if I'm lucky I have hepatitis. You have to help me."

He didn't know me, but I knew him by reputation. As a volunteer, patients had told me about their doctors, and this guy was known to be crazy, aggressive, and a fighter. I wanted him.

After looking at my records, he knew I was right, and we started doing tests. While the tests were being done, I was getting sicker and sicker, and everyone close to me was saying, "I'm sure everything is fine, don't worry." This was infuriating to hear. I knew something was wrong and no one was taking me seriously.

When all the test results were in, the doctor said, "Your liver is very bad."

"Is there a possible treatment?" I asked.

"Yes, there are a few things I can try."

"Can you ever get rid of it?"

"The literature says no, and I don't agree."

That was probably the nicest thing anyone ever said to me. He gave me hope. I knew people died from advanced liver mets. Once the cancer spreads to a major organ — it really doesn't matter which organ — it means the cancer has gone through your system.

He told me I had to have chemotherapy.

"How long will it take to lose my hair?" I asked.

"Two weeks from the day of your first treatment."

I immediately went down to order my wigs.

Besides the chemo, he put me on experimental megadoses of one of the killer drugs. This was in June, and I wasn't expecting to see the new year.

The drug had horrendous side effects. I got so weak I was unable to cover myself. I couldn't go to the bathroom alone. I couldn't get into the bathtub. I was either in bed at home or in the hospital. Once every three weeks I had the drug. Ten days later I was in hospital. Plus, one of the side effects of chemo is mouth sores. I had mouth sores in my mouth, down my throat, all over my tongue. There were big holes in my tongue. And I broke out in herpes all over my face. Then my saliva glands gave way, and saliva was pouring out of my mouth twenty-four hours a day. I had to hold a towel under my chin. I was a mess, yet sort of happy. If this drug was doing so much damage to me, then maybe it was also killing the cancer. Some patients hate the chemo, and I tell them, "Chemo is not the enemy, cancer is the enemy."

After four and a half months, my body got a little stronger. I was able to get three or four days of quality time out of my three-week cycle. I could actually do normal things, like go to a restaurant with a friend and have a salad. You have no idea how good normal things can feel.

Next I had surgery to take biopsies from my liver. Amazingly, my liver was clear. Now the doctor suggested doing a bone marrow transplant.

I said to him, "I know it's a risky procedure, does anyone really die in that room?"

"Yes."

I sort of knew the answer, but I thought he'd say, Yes, but it's never happened here, or Yes, but it's one in a million, but he just said, "Yes."

"You mean I could go in that room and not come out?"

"Yes."

Still, the transplant gave me hope. Theoretically my liver was clear but I knew the cancer was going to come back, and a bone marrow transplant could give me some extra time.

Before the transplant, I was meticulous in my preparations. I was getting myself ready, determined to be in good spirits by the time I checked into hospital. I made computer signs for my door. "I require privacy now." "Please don't enter." When I was taking a bath, I didn't want the doctors to come in. With the head nurse's permission, I put a notice in the front of my chart stating my requests. I asked the staff to call me Elaine. I'm Elaine to everybody, even to my kids' friends. I asked that my head be covered at all times. In the hospital I wore a turban and didn't want to be left without it if I was in a coma. I asked them to please close the door and the curtains at the appropriate times. I asked them that I be the first person to be informed of any changes in my condition.

I also wrote that my daughter wanted to be called, day or night, if there was something new, and I left her phone number. I bought Rubbermaid boxes in which to store my things in hospital so they wouldn't collect dust. I printed out the words of some very corny songs that had meaning to me, like "Climb Every Mountain," "I Believe," "You'll Never Walk Alone." I wanted that kind of spirit to go in with. I really planned it.

I bought a case of toilet paper so the kids wouldn't run out at home. They had power of attorney over my bank account, my safety deposit box, my living will. The more I prepared, the readier I became to leave. I cooked and baked and put everything into little Ziploc containers, one-person servings. My upright freezer was filled with food. When I first got sick, my daughter was with me a lot, and my son was home and lost weight. This way he could throw the ready-made food into the microwave. There were soups, cakes, meat, you name it. Every time I made another batch of something, I felt good. And every time I put the containers in, I felt good. I did what I could to leave everything in as much order as possible.

Before the transplant, I even went to see my rabbi. In Judaism, if the angel of death is coming down for someone, you try and hide the person by giving him a new first name. I said to the rabbi, "Remember, if I run into trouble, I'd like a new name, and if I die, I want a simple eulogy."

He came to see me in the hospital before the procedure and asked, "Do you want me to do your name?"

I said, "Yeah."

Now my first name is Chai Haimtov. Chai means life.

First I had the bone marrow harvest, where they take out your bone marrow and put it in the freezer. Then, before the transplant, they chemoed me to death with megadoses for five days to burn out every cell in the body, good and bad. I got weaker and weaker, I was almost at death's door, and then they put me in isolation and gave me back half of my bone marrow to try and stimulate growth again. After this procedure, people are usually in isolation for three weeks. I was in there for two months because my white blood counts and neutrophils were not rising fast enough. My bone marrow had had such a beating from all the treatments that it just wasn't multiplying. Plus I had a reaction to every medication they gave me. I shook in convulsions five or six times a day.

In the transplant room, I learned a lot about dignity. Before, I was very worried about losing dignity. But what matters is how you're treated. During the transplant period, you lose control, you have diarrhea, you don't make the washroom, and it's not important. The staff was absolutely wonderful, and I was never made to feel like I didn't have dignity. So I re-evaluated my definition of the word.

When my father was sick, I couldn't bear to see that he had lost his dignity. I think he had the beginnings of Alzheimer's, and he became a feeble little boy. I didn't like him like that. And I know my son, Aaron, can't stand to see me as the feeble little woman. I used to think he was angry at me for being sick. He almost couldn't look at me. Aaron will help and be good to me, but sometimes, when I'm particularly weak, he'll become impatient and curt. At first I couldn't understand it. Then one day I remembered I had been angry at my father because he wasn't the strong father I once knew.

My daughter is a very warm and affectionate person, but she almost has nothing physical to do with me since I'm sick. Her way of protecting herself is to keep a certain physical distance. If she gets too close to me, it'll be that much harder for her to lose me. But she lets me talk about anything I want. We've even discussed a death notice announcement. We've discussed eulogies. I told her I don't want to be made into St. Elaine. But she doesn't hold me, kiss me, touch me. She held my hand at a couple of high-stress points and that's it. Before we were kissy, huggy, warm. Aaron, who certainly doesn't let me touch him in public, has given me more physical warmth, though not a lot. He's come to the hospital and put his arms around me. Monica gives me much more time, and he gives me physical attention. I didn't understand all this at first. I had to work it out.

When I'm in the recovery room, Monica stands at the door, peeking in, waiting for me to open my eyes. You're not allowed to be there, but she's learned to push her way around a bit. She's a social worker, she knows you have to be aggressive. But she's not a social worker, she's my child and I'm her mother, and part of her is a child whose mother has cancer. We come home from the hospital, and she carries my bag up the stairs because I'm not allowed to carry, and then she sits down and says, "What's for supper?"

And I go and make supper, and she sits there watching me. We're both happy to go back to our old roles, where I'm the mother and she's the kid.

But my daughter should be out doing fun things, not sitting day after day in a transplant room or curled up in the hospital on a bed or sleeping in a chair. I feel like I'm a burden. She's young, and she should be enjoying her engagement, and I've burdened her. I wouldn't have felt that way about Peter. The normal, nice Peter would have taken care of me.

My mother is quite normal about my illness, as normal as you can be. At the beginning I had to force her to say the word cancer. Now she tells strangers that her daughter has cancer.

"I can't believe what's coming out of my mouth," she says. "Before I couldn't say the word, now I tell everybody. Someone on the bus says, "Gee, it's a nice day out," and I say, "Yes, and I'm going to see my daughter in the hospital."

And she tells them the whole story. She had a hard time when I got out of the hospital. For the three and a half months I was in there, she lost her life.

I kept saying, "Ma, you don't have to come every minute."

And she'd say, "There is nothing else that's important to me but being here."

As a mother I understand that, I would do the same. But I feel very sad about it. My mother should be enjoying the later years of her life, and she's not. Since I got sick, she hasn't gone away for the winter. She sold her place in Florida. And she doesn't do anything because I'm sick. All she wants to do is take care of me. When I got out of the hospital, she didn't know what to do with herself.

I called her regularly to ask, "What did you do today?"

"Nothing."

And she got a little older. She's seventy-four, cute, and not an old lady at all. But she aged in those three and a half months.

I never asked myself, Why me?

·Why not me? Why you? Why anybody? Now I'm going through why me? Since I started to be successful and all the people around me are dying. There were thirty people in that first experimental study. I was probably the worst off, and I'm clear. Most of the others are dead. Why does one person with the same disease respond to one drug and the other doesn't? I think about this every time one of my buddies dies. Every time a twenty-year-old kid on my floor dies, I ask myself, What did I do differently? Why am I alive?

I feel almost like the people who survived the concentration camps. There is a lot of guilt. I am deserting my kids. I was supposed to babysit with the grandchildren. And I'm destroying my poor mother. I speak to my friends and hear the sadness in their voices. I have made an entire circle of people sad.

Yes, I have the fighting spirit, which is important, otherwise they would have stopped treatment a long time ago. And I have a doctor who didn't say, She's going to die anyway, let's save the money on the drug.

And I've had support. Every time the rabbi came to see me, he told me they did a special prayer for me. That gave me strength. I needed lifts to and from the hospital every day. My friends were lining up, I'll take you Tuesday, I'll take you Wednesday. You can't do this alone.

As much as I think you have to fight, you also have to know when it's time. And you have to accept it. When I thought I was dying, I could handle it. But when I thought my son would graduate from university and I won't be there, and my kids will have children and I won't experience that part of their life, I couldn't bear it. But the dying part is not the problem. There's a leaving and a going. They're two separate issues. I'm not afraid to go, but the leaving is hard.

My daughter once asked me if I would like to die at home. It sounds very romantic. I think it's a horrendous thing to put on your children. Should they be alone when I die, without medical staff to come in and offer support? No. My father died in the hospital. A dying person needs certain physical things like bed pans, needs to be lifted, rolled, carried. Should that be their responsibility? I want them to be able to call the nurse when they need something. Let them just be there and we can mourn together. The nurses can do what they have to do.

☙

These days I have a lot of time to think, to figure things out. And sometimes, when I think of the end, I also think of the beginning, the beginning of the cancer. The first cancer I believe was caused by the horrible last five years of my marriage. And the depression and sadness I had for that year and a half after Peter left caused the spread. I had tremendous anger, none of it was at this illness. I had tremendous anger at the separation. I had invested in Peter. I gave him my life, and when I finally needed him, he left me and left my kids to bear the burden of me. I was very, very angry, anger that I didn't have anywhere to put. Now, I feel sorry for him because he must be doing his own suffering since the business went bankrupt.

With the bankruptcy I lost my group insurance plan. That was very frightening because I never want my treatment to be less aggressive because we can't afford certain drugs. Healthcare pays for some treatments, they don't pay for others. One year it cost me $13,000 for a certain drug, and my insurance paid for it. Thank God I'm not on it now! One year my drugstore bill was $325 every three weeks. The medication for my mouth was very expensive. It's scary.

My son said to me, "I feel sorry for Daddy. He ruined his life and he doesn't know it."

But now my daughter is getting married, and I'm still here. I feel lucky to be alive for the wedding, and I'm going to enjoy every minute of it. I'm enjoying every minute of the planning.

Now he's not watching the wedding preparations and he's not opening the RSVP cards. So he has a little chick. In three and a half years, my kids have never met the little chick. They've never been to his house. When he was driving the Jag and living like a king, he looked like the winner, and I was really angry. Now, I'm not sure if he's the winner. I don't know what he won.

After we got married and we bought our house, Peter said, "Now I'll never have to move again."

In his twenty-one years, he had moved twenty times. Since he left me, he's moved four times in three and a half years. He's also with someone who is just like his mother. And I remember soon after we met he said to me, "My mother is a witch. She's everything I don't want in a woman."

Peter wanted warmth, affection, things he didn't have at home. He's now with someone who works in a bank, is quite cold, and never smiles. He went full circle. There are pictures of Peter when he was small, tied to a tree. His mother was afraid to leave him out alone, and she had to wash the floor every third hour. He used to say to her, "Why don't you take me outside to play and stop cleaning the house?"

Yet the biggest criticism he had of me was that I was not the perfect housekeeper. I'm not a bad housekeeper, but sometimes there was a basket of laundry that didn't get folded. And in the last five years of the marriage, I could do nothing right.

His girlfriend is thirty-three, and I'm surprised she hasn't left him yet because things are not the way they were. The first year he left they went on twelve trips. He pissed away more money in that one year than he ever did in the whole marriage. Now he's not spending that kind of money, he's scared to death. I don't know how much money he has. I hope he has enough to invest or go into something else because as of last week, he's unemployed, and I'm dependent on this man.

I want to stay alive as long as I have a shred of hope and a shred of quality to my life. I suspect the definition of quality changes as you get sicker, and what you once thought wasn't quality becomes quality, just like what you think is old isn't so old when you get there. I guess that changes like my vision of dignity.

When I first got sick, I felt everything could still be fixed. I still wanted whole and perfect. Then you reach a point where you can't fix it all, it's never going to be what it was. Life will never be what it was, your body will never be what it was, and you start accepting less and less and less. Before I liked perfection, I liked everything to fit, everything had to be even, two cars and two garages, and then we had four cars. Now things don't fit anymore. I don't fit anymore. I don't have the husband and I don't have the health, but it's okay. You no longer expect things to fit, so it doesn't have to be perfect, so it's less than perfect, so it's much less than perfect, so it's much, much less than perfect. You keep settling and settling, and then you don't even mind settling.

I used to put makeup on every day because there might be a blemish or a mark. Now it's just blush and finish. I don't go around looking like I've got cancer, but I don't have to be perfect either. Before the separation, I was never perfect enough, but I kept trying. Now I do my best and that's it.

If I still had my perfect-four family life, would I be able to accept the end, or did I already accept "the family torn and the life broken" with the broken marriage? If I would still have my perfect world, I would be fighting the diagnosis. This way I am fighting the disease. I accept the diagnosis. Before, I had tried to hold on to my marriage when it was really falling apart. And when I had breast cancer and the doctor said chemotherapy was not the required treatment for minimal cancer, I listened to him and did nothing. In my heart, I was afraid to lose my hair because I would be less perfect than I already was. By then I knew Peter didn't really like me, and he would have liked me even less without hair. If I had been separated at that point, would I have been brave enough to ask for chemotherapy, even though they were not giving it?

This is rough stuff down here on earth. I think the place up there has got to be terrific because we couldn't have been created for this. Sometimes I think, Boy, I'm going to have a good party up there. I'm going to be in such good company. I've befriended so many people as a volunteer and as a patient, and so many have died. I've been to so many funerals.

I always knew I was dying. I accepted that two years ago and then took on the bonuses. In those two years, I've spent a tremendous amount of time in the hospital. Some people would say, was that worth it?

The day before the wedding, I went to a car wash and got a very bad headache, which is unusual for me. I had made this fancy basket to put in the kids' hotel room so they could have some goodies when they checked in. As I was driving it downtown to the hotel, my arm started to go cold. I thought it might be the air conditioning. When I arrived, I couldn't take the key out of the ignition. My right hand didn't work. A guy from the hotel had to carry the basket in for me. I asked for a card to write a note. I couldn't hold the pen steady enough. The girl at the desk had to write it for me.

I got back in my car and said, "What do I do?"

I was due to go for a manicure appointment. My hand was getting better so I went, and by the time I got there my hand was perfect. But I was nervous. After the manicure, I drove to the hospital. They gave me a neurological examination, and the resident said, "I don't find anything wrong with you."

"I don't think you've made me very happy." Really, I would have liked them to find a stroke.

They arranged to run a scan, and as I sat there waiting I thought, I don't want the results.

I found the resident and said, "I think I should go home. My daughter is getting married tomorrow. I'll come back Monday."

I went home and didn't tell anyone. The next day, Sunday, I was perfect. The wedding was perfect, the weather was perfect, everything was perfect. It was a happy, relaxed, joyous day, not marked by illness. I was surrounded by my family and friends, people who cared about me. I walked through the door alone and saw all these people smiling at me. I felt good. It was hard to walk down the aisle alone. I walked down halfway and Peter walked down halfway. He didn't bring the girlfriend, which made it easier. But, really, I didn't need him anymore.

Monday morning I couldn't get out of bed, my body was so exhausted. By Tuesday I had dizzy spells. Wednesday I went to a meeting at the hospital and my head was spinning. Thursday I was so dizzy with headaches I couldn't move. Friday I went for my treatment at the hospital and the doctor gave me a neurological examination. I was sure it was brain mets. Friday night I had a scan and the results were what I expected. The moment that arm went numb I said, "Dear God, no."

I asked the doctor, "Do you have any experimental therapy up your sleeve?"

He said, "I'm thinking, I'm thinking."

I love my doctor, I know this man will run to the end of the earth if there is a drop of a chance that he can do something for me.

On Monday he presented his plan. It was totally experimental, high risk, never been done before. He said I can die on the table or come out a potato. I grabbed it. Go for broke. I had no illusion about what he was offering. I wasn't expecting a miracle, but doing something is better than doing nothing. The object was to put chemo through my groin into my brain, not knowing if I would stroke or hemorrhage, and try it. Chemo doesn't scare me. I love chemo, it's an ammunition.

When I agreed to the procedure, he was as happy as a lark, and that was okay. If they can learn something and ten guys down the road can benefit from this, then that gives my life more meaning.

As soon as they diagnosed the brain mets, I was given steroids. The steroids take away the dizziness and headaches, but they also cause a lot of trouble. I'm up during the night and I'm falling off my feet during the day. A healthy person would have trouble functioning with the hours I'm sleeping. The steroids also make me look like Mama Cass. I can't wear anything but sweatsuits. Nothing with a waist fits me. My neck and face have ballooned. And I'm growing hair on my face. Hair! Me, who runs for electrolysis if I have three blond hairs. But I'm not going to get hung up about it. Three and a half years ago, the marks on my breast felt so degrading. Now I'm no longer there.

As a cancer patient, you get advance notice before you die. You generally know you have X number of months before the end. Suddenly, with this experimental procedure, I could be dead from one day to the next. That was a little mind-boggling, if I can die in one day, on the table, what am I supposed to be doing in the meantime?

I thought, what else can I do for the children in the few weeks I have left? I put a letter with my will saying I would like the kids to put aside a little money for the grandchildren's birthdays so they can be acknowledged by me. I also wrote in my will that my kids should always be close and never let anything come between them. And they should take care of my mother. I kept thinking, Is there something else?

I was worried that I never gave Monica my recipes, and my kids liked my cooking and baking and they'll never be able to duplicate it. I wrote out all my recipes, since a lot are in my head. I've given them all to my daughter and now she can make all the things I used to make. It's comforting to know my things will be carried on.

I was also worried about my belongings. What was going to happen to them? My daughter doesn't have my taste. My son would rent an apartment and have his own things. What are you going to do, have a garage sale? I pictured all my belongings on the driveway, and I was heartbroken. That was bothering me a lot. We talked about it, and I didn't say they should give everything away, because they need the money, but I said that maybe the people close to me can have certain things of mine they want and sell the rest.

I also asked myself, What could I say for the next thirty years that I won't be here? Then I go to my daughter's house and see my influence. I watch her do things, I look at the brands of food she buys, and she doesn't know that I'm in that house. It gives me such pleasure. And I know when she'll be a mother, she'll be the same kind of mother I was. And I know that in the last twenty years I've probably given whatever is possible to give, and what they didn't yet get I wouldn't be able to give. So I guess my job is done.

I feel awful about Aaron. He's twenty-one and doesn't have a close relationship with his father. He's a bright boy with a good future, and he has a sister who has been a mother to him her whole life, so I know he'll be okay, but how can I not feel I'm deserting the ship?

My mother spent her whole life giving, and I would have liked to know that when she is sick and old and dying I could be there for her. My daughter has lupus and will have a high-risk pregnancy, and I remember saying to her, "When you have children I'll help you, I'll take care of you." Hey, where am I going?

❦

The procedure for brain mets was over four hours long, and I came through it really well. Now I have to go for two weeks of radiation. I'm back to cooking and baking. I get some really tired spells, but I'm functional.

The doctors don't give me a time frame and I don't ask. I find that very unproductive. If I know I'm terminal, I don't want to think time. My farthest expectation is that maybe I'll have many months of decent quality. I already had a two-year extension on my life, two years I wasn't supposed to have. And I enjoyed every minute, and I will continue to enjoy it. For some reason, I'm not depressed. I think I should be, but I'm not.

Since I was diagnosed with brain mets, I've lost all my credibility. People are waiting for a neurological sign, waiting for me to say or do something wrong. I feel a lot of pressure to prove I don't have a neurological problem. Normally I'm a crazy person, I like to act crazy, do crazy things, and now I'm afraid to do that. Of course, I'm also worried that I will have neurological signs and check myself every four minutes.

Other than my separation, I have no major regrets. I never had big demands in life, so I have no disappointments. I never had any grandiose schemes. I've never been envious. I've never wanted what someone else had. I didn't have that kind of turmoil. I've always known how to make me happy in my way. I was very fulfilled. My three years as a volunteer at the hospital probably gave more meaning to my life than I've ever had. I know I helped a lot of people through some hard times.

On Friday I was on the ward the whole day, and the nurses dragged me from room to room. Could you see this one? That one can use you. And there were three volunteers on the floor, but none have had cancer, and it makes a difference. Because of the cancer, I'm much more valuable. At the end of the day, when I got into my car, I was physically and mentally wiped, but I felt so good. When you have been given an extended lease on life, you want meaning to it, and there is such a good feeling knowing you did something worthwhile. If I can help someone get through the hour, I feel rewarded.

I'm really not superstitious, but since I'm sick I have a blue Rubbermaid box filled with little things people have given me. Whatever I get for good luck, I keep. A friend just came back from Italy, and she brought me a little plaque of St. Somebody-or-other, a help saint. She said, "I know it's not your thing, but I couldn't resist."

I said, "I'll take it."

I have a Buddha, an elephant, a turtle from Japan that promises health and long life. This is so not me, but since I'm sick I'm collecting everything people give me. And this box comes with me every time I go into hospital.

I was in for a second procedure, same as the first, this time to the other side of the head. But they had kept postponing the date because they were waiting for my platelets to rise. If your platelet count is low, you can hemorrhage. You don't want to be in an accident because you could bleed to death. Platelet counts should be between 140 and 440. At one time mine was as low as four, and it was under twenty for eight months. They don't know how I was able to drive and run around.

The second procedure was harder on me. Because of all the drugs I was taking, my system went crazy. I was running a 103-degree fever and had to stay in hospital for three weeks. My sister came for a visit and became hysterical. She said to me, crying, "How could this be you?"

She was remembering me the way I was. I was a live wire, and suddenly there I was, weak and sick. She got so upset, and I realized she was just seeing it for the first time. When it happens slowly, you don't really see it. Suddenly, she saw the deterioration of my life.

Next I'll have to have tests to check if the cancer is in the nervous system. If you can have worse than brain mets, it can be in the nervous system.

I'm weak and I don't like it. Every time I have some energy, I go and do some cooking or baking. I have seen a lot of patients give up. My platelets were dropping again last week. And yesterday I was so low, no energy, and I used to be a super-high-stamina person. I was so frustrated I burst out crying. I want to drive the car to get what I want. But I can't, I need people to drive me around. Everyone is doing errands for me. And my car is dirty. I can't stand a dirty car, and I can't ask someone to take me to get the car washed. Really, if I would have a different personality, I would have given up already.

But, you know, I have never felt it would be easier to give up. Never, never, never. There was a time when I wouldn't have thought I had the strength to fight cancer. I knew I was strong, but not when it came to health, the body. When I got breast cancer, I wondered, How can I go through with this? After a while the answer came to me: With dignity. And that's exactly what I've been doing, living and fighting with dignity.

I'm not yet ready to die, but I'm prepared to die. And I'm not at all afraid of dying. How can I be? Really, in my mind, I'm already dead. I have done what I've needed to do, and what I would still like to do there is no more time for, so now they're only flickering thoughts with no substance. And soon even the flickers will be extinguished.

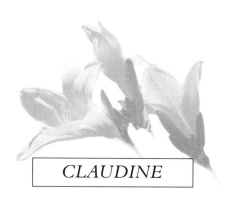

CLAUDINE

Claudine was a thirty-five-year-old AIDS victim. Keith, whose portrait begins on page 169, gave me her name. When I called her and told her about my project, she immediately agreed to be interviewed, saying that the end of her life was not something she could talk about with her family and friends. She welcomed the opportunity to review her life.

She asked that the interviews be at my house, since she was still well enough to travel around the city, and it was summer, the weather was pleasant. She sounded as if she welcomed the chance to go somewhere.

Claudine was tall and slim, with a dancer's body. Her long, dark brown hair fell around her face in curls. She said she had dyed her hair numerous outrageous colours, but now she was leaving it natural. She had toned down her once-flamboyant style, but her original exotic flair was still evident in the way she dressed.

Her voice was clear, strong, rooted within the self. She was always in a reflective, positive mood. She carefully thought about some of my questions before giving her answers.

She welcomed the opportunity to go deeper into her life, to search for answers she might not have thought of before, to see her life in totality.

CʒƐ

In retrospect I'm happy to have lived all this. It has helped me to appreciate life from a totally different perspective. It has opened my eyes to the present. And if today a cure were found for AIDS, I don't think I would take it. I've grown too used to living with the virus. I was twenty-seven when I found out I had it. Now I'm thirty-five and have arrived at a point where I no longer think about next month or even next week. If all of a sudden I were told I could live to the age of eighty, I would panic. What would I do with my life? I'm too used to living with the idea of death. For me death has become a source of comfort. It has also added a greater intensity to life.

I have never before been as aware of people, myself, and life as I am now. Before, I was constantly doing things. I never stopped to think. I didn't feel alive because I didn't think of being alive. Now I have acquired a profound love of life because I've confronted death. First my husband's and then my own. It seems sad that one needs an illness and the death of a loved one to appreciate life.

Nine years ago, Alex and I were trying to have a baby. A year later, he wasn't feeling well. One Friday I came home from work and started to prepare supper, expecting him to arrive soon. The phone rang. It was Alex telling me he was in the hospital. I said, "Of course, you told me you were going in for some tests."

He said, "I've already had the tests."

"Did they find out what's wrong?"

"Yes."

"So you can come home now."

"It would be better if I stayed here a bit longer."

"Why?"

"Because they're not sure."

"Have they identified the problem or haven't they?"

"Yes. They found the problem. They're almost sure."

"Well, what is it?"

"They think I have AIDS." Said in a monotone. Flat.

My hand with the phone in it just dropped by my side. Panic. Paralysis. Then I picked up the phone again.

"Tell me it's not true. It's true."

"I've been wanting to talk to you about it since December."

I was shocked. "If you had any doubts, why didn't you say something? Do something? I must have it as well."

"Yes, probably." Still the monotone. No emotion. "You have to get tested immediately."

"I don't believe it. There's been a mistake. Ask for another test."

"They've already done all sorts of tests, and it's definitely AIDS. I even have pneumonia and have to stay in hospital."

"What are you going to do?"

"I'll come back to the house, pick up some things, and write out the rent cheque."

I put down the phone and went hysterical. It was the end of my world. No children. Alex will die. And I loved him. He's the only person I have ever loved. Until he arrived, I kept pacing up and down the apartment like a caged animal. I felt on the edge of insanity. The walls were undulating before my eyes.

It was strange because I know the homosexual community very well. Most of my friends are gay. A friend's brother died of AIDS a few years back. But I never thought AIDS could touch me. It seemed so far from my reality. I knew Alex had relations with men, but he protected himself. The AIDS virus was not a part of our lives.

Alex arrived. I immediately said, "Tell me it's not true. Tell me you didn't call me."

"It's true." And he sat down at the kitchen table to write out the rent cheque. He said, "Claudine, I'm going to die, and I don't know how much time I have left."

He was very calm. I continued pacing up and down, saying, "It's not true, it's not true."

He said, "Yes, it is. And I'm glad I'm going to die. I'll never forgive myself for having given this to you. All because I went outside of our relationship."

I couldn't even take him in my arms. I didn't even touch him. I felt like I was watching a play. Like I had left my body. I saw the whole scene from on top. The pain. The incredulity. Alex went to pack a small bag and left. I was so numb I couldn't even go with him to the hospital. I stayed at home and cried the whole night. The next day, I went to see him. I found out the AIDS was quite advanced, and he had to stay in hospital for a month.

The following Monday, I went to get tested. A week later, I got the results. Till the moment I got them I was certain I didn't have it. The doctor called to say I was HIV positive. It was a total surprise, like I had been wearing blinkers. But I was still in good health. My blood count was relatively high. My only thought was to remain healthy till Alex died. I was certain that would happen within weeks.

While Alex was in the hospital, I was emotionally on hold. I was working full time plus taking care of his needs. There was no time for anything else.

When he came back home, I began to live a nightmare. It was too difficult to get used to the idea that we both had it. Our families were always calling us, "How are you?"

I just wanted to escape while their questions kept pulling me back to reality. Every time we saw his parents, they wanted to discuss the funeral arrangements. We told them we didn't want to talk about it. They kept insisting. Soon after Alex came out of the hospital, our fridge broke and we bought a new one. His parents said, "Why are you bothering to buy new appliances? You're going to die soon anyway."

Alex went back to work, and he was fine for a while. We went to Jamaica for a week to relax and try to forget about what was happening. When we got back, we began to talk about the illness. The more we talked, the more our relationship developed and grew. Since we had no idea how long we had left, we decided to spend as much time together as possible, to live everything to the fullest. We went to exhibitions, plays, ballets, concerts, operas, films, everything. We still continued to do what we did before, we just did more of it and were together more often. Also, from that point on, Alex didn't go with another man.

I began to buy books on AIDS to try to understand the illness. We discussed what could happen, what sort of illnesses we could develop. Alex said, "I can have about three pneumonias before I die. I've had one, I can have two more." Our perspective was very concrete and objective, centred on the physical aspects of the illness.

Then I went through a phase of being really angry at the virus. Angry at Alex for not having talked to me about it when he first noticed the symptoms. I am a fairly strong character and a fighter. I say what I think. I'm not careful. I kept asking, "Why didn't you say anything before? Why didn't you confide in me?" I think I goaded him.

He said he was in denial. He was so afraid he had AIDS that he didn't want to talk about it. He thought talking about it was going to concretize it, make it real.

Sexually, the relationship changed. Besides the practical difficulties of making love, we couldn't kiss again till the day he died. Alex constantly had thrush in his mouth, and if we French kissed he could give it to me. I kissed him on the cheeks and on the lips, but not a French kiss. We couldn't have oral intercourse because he could give me a yeast infection from his mouth. Once we tried it and I did get a yeast infection.

The first seven or eight months, we tried to make love as before. And we couldn't. I was scared of getting pregnant because I had stopped taking the pill. Plus we were both afraid that Alex would give me more of the virus. Every time we tried to make love I saw death on top of me. It was hard. When you've spent over ten years making love, you develop certain habits, and you automatically try to revert to the old pattern. And it's frustrating when you find it no longer works. For a while we couldn't make love. Then we began to use condoms. That was another problem. We had never used them before and were both nervous that the condom would break. Penetration was a problem.

But we were constantly in touch with each other, talking about and analyzing what was going on. One day, during one of our discussions, after a particularly frustrating attempt at trying to make love, we decided we had to find a different way of doing it. We learned to touch each other more, caress each other, hold each other, give each other massages. Our physical contact became more sensual and less sexual.

For a while, I was still in good health, and then my blood count dropped to 200 and I was put on medication. When I began the medication, I was furious. I always had to force myself to take it. I hate pills. I had never taken anything before in my life, not even for menstrual cramps. The pills were a constant reminder of the fact that I was sick. Plus I had all sorts of side effects. That made me even more angry. Finally I told myself to stop fighting it. The pills might help and allow me to stay relatively healthy while Alex was still alive.

Eight months after his diagnosis Alex again landed in hospital. From that point on, he became weaker and weaker. Life changed gradually. We did less. We no longer went cross-country skiing. We no longer did sports. We went to films, plays, concerts and talked a lot.

I said, "If you're better today we'll go for a walk. If you're not nauseous, we'll go to a restaurant."

Two years after diagnosis, he began to deteriorate quickly. And he was again admitted to hospital for a month. This was his second pneumonia. When he came back home, we had to install an apparatus around the bathtub so he could get in and out on his own. Inside the apartment, he walked around with a cane. He needed a wheelchair to go outside. Now he was so weak that I had to do everything. I worked a full day, then came home and made supper. I cleaned the house. I did the shopping and laundry for both of us. I felt like a maid. But I loved Alex so much. I would have done anything for him.

He did what he could. When he was well he took care of the bills from his chair. He took care of his funeral arrangements because he didn't want me to have problems with his family after he died.

By now he was a totally changed person physically. It had happened gradually, but there were always changes. Each morning I was confronted by a very morbid reality. I saw Alex nude every day. He had Kaposi's sarcoma all over his body. He had lost his hair because of the chemotherapy. He had become very thin, and at the same time his stomach, eyes, and penis were terribly swollen. He was in such pain that we couldn't even have sex. He had diarrhea. He vomited.

He couldn't hold down his food. It was hard for me to see someone I loved go through such a metamorphosis. Plus I was convinced that after Alex's death the same things were going to happen to me.

I took care of Alex, and I was curious. It was strange. When he developed something new, I consulted all the books I had bought to figure out what AIDS was. We discussed it. I carefully examined every new spot, I outlined it in ink, and a week later looked at it again to see if it had grown. I went with him to see the doctor and asked what could be done about this or that. I developed a medical curiosity about his symptoms. At the same time, I carefully watched my own body, scrutinizing every area for new developments. I wanted to know what was happening. What does this virus do to the body? Of course, I also thought, I better learn everything I can now before my turn comes around.

Alex didn't mind my inspection, but he was basically sad throughout the illness, sad that he had given this to me. He sometimes said, "Don't worry, I'm going to die soon. I know I'm useless. I'm just a weight on you. Soon you'll be free of me." It was a bit of emotional blackmail.

Sometimes I could put up with what was going on, and sometimes my anger against the illness would flare up. Evidence of it was everywhere. I couldn't get away from it. The wheelchair was in the hallway. Every time I went to hang up my coat I had to walk around it. There were pills in the kitchen, in the bathroom. I'm a very clean and organized person, and the apartment always looked like a mess, filled with things that seemed out of place.

Two and a half years after the initial diagnosis, Alex went into hospital with his third pneumonia. We both knew this was it. His lungs were filled with Kaposi's sarcoma. He was totally swollen. He had no more feeling in his fingers or toes. And he continued to deteriorate from the moment he entered the hospital. He never complained, never cried. When he had been in the hospital before, we had always talked about what was happening to his body. We analyzed what the doctor had said, tried to find the best treatment for new symptoms. This time we didn't talk about the illness at all. We talked of our love, about the times we had spent together, the past.

I stopped working and spent full time with him at the hospital. I slept there every night on a fold-out cot beside him. I totally forgot about myself. My full attention was on him. I helped to feed him. Read books or articles to him. I put on his favourite cassettes. Also, I knew it was important for him that I always arrive in a good mood, well dressed, fully made up. That took some effort. Every day, when I went home to take a shower or bath, I cried my eyes out.

This time things were so difficult for me that I developed a case of shingles. My arms and chest were full of small red blisters that broke open. All these blisters followed the course of a nerve so they were incredibly painful and they burned. Besides my regular medication, I now had to take various painkillers. But my sole interest was to keep myself together till Alex died. To be there for him.

Alex wanted to speak with people individually before he died. He asked me to organize it so that he could speak with one person a night. Though he was in terrible pain and his body was now totally deformed by the illness, he was fully lucid and logical. One night he spoke to a good friend of his. Another night it was my brother-in-law, then my sister, then my two nephews together. Everything he said was very specific to each person. And people had to listen to him because they knew he was dying. He told his sister, Nadine, to take her life into her own hands. He told his parents what he thought about them and how he felt about how they had raised him. He told them they had paid no attention to him as he was growing up, they had rejected him, and they're doing the same thing with Nadine. He told them to take care of her, to be more tolerant, and not to always impose their view of life. Alex's parents don't really like their children. They want them to like what they like, hunting, fishing, hockey. They can't accept that different people have different tastes.

I was the last one he spoke to. To me he mostly spoke about love. He said, "I hope you won't suffer as I have, but you'll see, death isn't that terrible."

He expected me to follow him soon after he died, so he told me to enjoy the time I have left. Work less, live more. He told me to think of myself, to spoil myself, make new friends. He said, "You'll just have enough money, but with the little you have, enjoy life. If you need anything extra, your mother will be there for you."

One day, after he had been in hospital for a month, he said, "I know this is the end, but I don't want to leave you."

I said, "I don't want you to go."

But he was terribly ill.

Later the doctor took me aside and said, "You must tell him you're willing to let him go. He's suffering too much and only hanging on because of you."

After that I went home. Took a bath. And thought about what the doctor had said. Maybe he's right.

I went back to the hospital. That night, just before Alex fell asleep, I said, "I don't want you to die, but I can't see you like this anymore. It's too difficult. I want you to feel free to go. You will die and live something more beautiful. You'll see a light that will be warm and loving, allow yourself to embrace the light."

He said, "You want me to go."

I said, "I love you. I want you to be with me but in health. I don't want to see you this sick."

He said, "I don't want to leave you. You're the one I love most in the world."

I said, "You're the one I love most in the world, too."

He fell asleep, and I went to sleep beside him on the cot. A little later he woke me up, saying, "It's the end. I'm about to die. I'm going to let myself go."

I got up to be beside him. I asked, "Can you see the light?"

"Yes."

"Go toward the light. It'll get bigger and bigger the closer you get. And you're going to feel wonderful."

He took a deep breath and then stopped breathing. I put my hand in front of his mouth to feel if there was any air. He opened his eyes and said, "No, I'm not dead yet."

That was hard. I said, "Let yourself slide out of your body. Let it go. You'll feel light and free."

And he let himself go. I was holding his hand and I saw him leave. I saw a white and mauve mass rising, leaving his chest and forehead. And I kept saying, "Go toward the light." And I saw a cluster of little stars above him. As I watched, I was filled with such peace and happiness and had absolutely no physical or psychological pain. When this mass of white and mauve fully left his body, I thought, "That's it. He's gone." Then I started to cry. But I was very calm.

Alex and I had written out our will together, and we both asked to be cremated. Alex also specified that he be buried in a public place. He didn't want to spend money on a private plot. He wanted his burial to cost the minimum so I would have more money left to live on.

At the funeral, I didn't know which was worse, the psychological pain or the physical pain of the shingles. Also the numerous painkillers I was on made everything seem surreal. A week after the ceremony, his box of ashes was lowered into a hole, like a catacomb for little boxes. And his name was added to the plaque with the names of others who had already been buried there.

Three days later, Alex's mother called me, totally hysterical because she didn't want Alex buried with strangers. She wanted his box of ashes dug out from where it was, reburied in a plot that was to be bought in the cemetery, and when I died I could be buried next to him. She wanted me to pay $3,000 for the plot.

I said, "I'm not interested in spending $3,000 for a piece of land. Alex wanted to be where he is. We have to respect his wishes, not yours."

She said, "No, it was your wish to see him buried in the cheapest possible way."

I said, "This is in Alex's will. I don't want to discuss it."

Later she called my mother. She wouldn't stop. Finally I went to see her and said, "Listen, you can't think of Alex being underground. He's not down there. He's up there. Think of his soul, not his ashes. The ashes are nothing."

She was horrified.

After the funeral I spent one month on my mother's sofa, crying. Then I said to myself, I have to continue to live.

I embarked upon a life of activity. I visited my family in Switzerland, and while there I went into a nearby church. As soon as I entered, I immediately felt Alex's presence around me. I felt his soul really close to me and clearly heard him say, "Continue to live, continue to be happy."

After the trip, when I returned home to the apartment, I again felt Alex's energy, like an envelope around me. It was very soothing and comforting.

I said to him, "You can go now. I'll be all right alone." And I felt his soul leaving. But in a way I feel he has never left, he lives on within me.

A year after Alex's death, I began to work only three days a week. Soon I met Philip and we began to go out. Sexually it was perfect. There was a strong physical attraction between us. But I wanted him to be like Alex. And he was just the opposite. Alex was always very neat and I'm neat. When Philip took a shower there was water everywhere and he never wiped it up. He left his clothes all over the house. Plus we always did what I suggested. He never came up with any of his own ideas. If I said I wanted to see this film, fine. If I wanted to hear that concert, fine. He never presented an alternative possibility.

Two months into the relationship, I went off to Europe for three weeks. One week to Switzerland with my mother and two weeks on my own to Paris and Rome. Someone had once broken into my apartment, so I asked Philip to keep an eye on it while I was gone. I gave him my keys. I left him love notes everywhere. I sent him postcards.

One night, when I was alone in the hotel room in Italy, I again felt Alex's presence around me. I heard him say, "You just have one life, live it. Now is when you have to live, not when you're sick and dying."

I knew he was referring to Philip.

My sister and I had had a terrible fight over Philip when we began to go out. She kept accusing me of betraying Alex. I think she was jealous because she wasn't very happy with her own life. And she thinks I have no right to enjoy life or to be with anyone because I have AIDS. It doesn't occur to her that I might need some affection.

When I came back, Philip picked me up at the airport. As soon as we got home, I went straight to sleep. The next morning I was up at five. He was still asleep. I went to the bathroom barefoot and immediately stepped on something sharp and cut my foot. I didn't have my glasses on and couldn't see anything. I went back to the bedroom for my glasses and then I saw. He had broken a glass in the bathroom and the pieces were all over the floor. There were empty beer bottles everywhere. The bathtub was grey. I don't think he washed it in the three weeks he was there. After my shower I went to the kitchen. It was a mess. Then I went to see my plants. My African violets were dying. That was it. I screamed. I went into the bedroom, shook him awake and said, "Get up and go."

He said, "What's wrong?"

I said, "Don't you realize plants need to be looked after? They're living things."

He said, "You watered them before leaving."

"That was three weeks ago! And the broken glass in the bathroom? Didn't it occur to you to clean up the mess? Didn't it occur to you to wash the bathtub?" I was furious.

He got up, dressed, and left. But at least the time I had spent with him made me realize that I was able to have feelings for someone else besides Alex. I could have a sexual desire for another man. That was important for me.

The most difficult part of this illness is sexual relationships. As soon as I'm attracted to someone, I think, I'm going to have to tell him what I have. And it's so difficult that I think I'd be better off without a man in my life. I sublimate sex. I channel it into other things. When I told Philip, he finished off a bottle of Scotch and became totally drunk. A few days later, he came back, and we began to go out. I always feel I have to immediately tell them. Really, I should just begin the relationship and ask the man to protect himself. When the relationship begins to solidify, then I can tell him. Of course, then he's going to get angry that I didn't say anything earlier. But if I tell him immediately, it'll scare him off. That's happened to me several times.

My second experience with death was nearly four years after Alex died. My father had a fatal heart attack. His funeral was held at the same church as Alex's and with the same priest. Even the coffin was similar. Once again I saw Alex's funeral, and I cried and cried. Everybody came to comfort me, but I wasn't crying for my father, I was crying for Alex. When I went up to the open coffin, I touched his hand and thought, "We hardly had a relationship." Now he's dead and didn't even know I had AIDS. My mother hadn't wanted me to tell him. And he was told that Alex had died of cancer.

My father's death changed nothing in my life because I had never done anything with him. When I was in school, he never looked at my report card. He never came to any of my ballet performances. When I was nineteen, I left St. Jerome to live in Montreal, and he never came to see my apartment. When Alex was ill, he never came to visit him in the hospital. I wasn't at all certain that my father even loved me. I don't think he loved anyone except himself, money, and the cats.

My father was a hairdresser. In Switzerland he had had his own salon, where he gave treatments to people who were losing their hair or who had problems with greasy or dry hair. Then he had an almost fatal accident. He fell into a coma and was supposed to die. My mother took care of all the funeral arrangements. Suddenly my father came to. And when he was fully well he decided to move to Canada. He had the American Dream. But my father was never happy, never satisfied with where he was and what he had. When in Canada he always said it was better in Switzerland. When in Switzerland he said it was better in Canada. Here he set up a hair salon in the basement of our house. I was born a couple of years after they arrived in Quebec, when my sister was already fifteen years old and my mother was forty-four.

My mother's happiness was my sister and me. She did everything for us, does even today. My father was not at all affectionate with her. And she never showed any warmth toward him. She wanted a man just to have children. My mother was also a hairdresser and helped my father professionally. The two worked very hard together and made good money. But there was no love between them.

My mother is the opposite of my father. She has always been sociable. I inherited her capacity to enjoy life, her ability to look at the positive side of things, and her humour. My father was always sad, quiet, but very cultured and intelligent. You could talk to him about books, music, politics. We always had passionate discussions around the dinner table.

My parents were two women, my mother and sister, and they both spoiled me. I had everything I needed. Other children had one or two dolls. I had all the dolls on the market. I had dolls that could dance, eat, walk. I had a room full of toys. I was taken on trips. I didn't eat meat, so my mother always made me special meals. I never had to do any housework. I never helped with the dishes, ironing, or cooking. I had everything done for me. And I was given everything I wanted. My father gave me nothing. He paid no attention to me.

He wasn't interested in people unless they could give him money. He was always very nice to his customers, always polite, caring, interested. He asked them how they were, how their wives were. He remembered details about their lives. With us he couldn't care less. He showed no interest.

I always got my Christmas gifts in two stages. One set on Christmas Eve, on the twenty-fourth, when my father told me how much each gift cost, and the rest the following morning, when he was still asleep, because my mother and sister didn't want me to open them all in front of him. He always thought they bought me too many gifts. My father was a real miser. He bought nothing for us or the house. My sister, who lived with us till she was thirty-three, was a nurse and bought what we needed. If a lamp broke, she was the one to replace it. If we needed a new couch, she went out to buy it.

In the basement, where my father had his salon, I had a room with a sound system. One day he showed a client the whole basement, which had just been renovated. My sister had bought the carpet and all the furniture. As he was showing the client around, I was there with my earphones, listening to music. As the client came in, the record had just ended, and I heard my father say, "We found this carpet in someone's garbage can. We bought the furniture at a second-hand store for just a few dollars."

He didn't want the client to think he had money. I took off my earphones and said, "That's not true." I told the client we had bought the carpet in such and such a place and paid this much for it, the furniture cost so much, and went on to name the cost of every item. My father was furious.

I wasn't an easy child for my parents. I kicked my mother when she did something I didn't like or didn't give me what I wanted. I was terrible. Once my father showed me his hand to signal that he was going to hit me, and I did the same to him. When we sat down for dinner, I did all the talking. My father used to say, "Stop talking. You're always talking."

I talked a lot. I got very good marks in school, and the teachers always wrote on my report card, "A good student but talks too much." Alex told me I even spoke in my sleep.

When I was young, I was very argumentative. My father was the same way. He was nice to his customers, but with anyone else he was always ready for a fight. In those days I was very interested in politics and often got into political arguments. My father and I were always arguing. And I disagreed with him on purpose. My sister was the opposite of me. She was very docile, never answered back. She was always afraid to say what she thought. I think when I argued with my father a part of her liked it because I also spoke for her.

My mother and I had some pretty big fights as well. When I was an adolescent, she always thought I came home too late. She waited up for me in the living room and made a scene when I got in. Then didn't speak to me for a couple of days. It wasn't very pleasant. And on top of that, she was constantly afraid that I would have an argument with my father. She was always on edge, thinking, What is she going to say this time? After every argument, my father would get angry at her because he blamed her for my attitude.

I was twenty-four when I realized that arguing with my father wasn't going to get me anywhere. Bit by bit I stopped correcting him or defending my position, and I let him talk. When I changed my attitude toward him, my mother was able to relax and be supportive of me. Before, she was so afraid of having my father angry at her that she just couldn't be there for me emotionally. She could give me things, but there was no praise for anything. No interest in the things I tried to do.

Also, my mother never taught me anything. I was her little girl and she took me everywhere, but she never said, Come, I'll show you how to do this or that. When I started something, she never encouraged me. So I never finished anything. Even today it's hard for me to finish what I start. She knew how to sew very well and never taught me. Once I bought a simple pattern for a skirt. And she criticized everything I did. She was such a perfectionist. I never finished the skirt. When I asked my mother to show me how to cook something, she became impatient. She wasn't capable of teaching. My sister can't do anything in the kitchen, either. When my mother is at my house and I cook, it's a nightmare. Everything has to be done the way she does it. She refuses to see that there might be another way of doing something.

Almost everything I learned came from my sister. I saw her read and I wanted to do the same thing. She taught me to read when I was five years old. I was always reading. She liked opera and classical music. I also began to listen to music. When I was eight or nine she introduced me to all sorts of opera singers. But I always lacked self-confidence because of my parents. I had good grades but never got any encouragement or praise. They never told me I was pretty. When I was young I decided to take ballet lessons, and though my mother paid for them, she never showed any excitement after one of my performances.

I don't know if it was because of my background, but early on I realized I didn't act or think like other people around me. I didn't quite fit in. And I was drawn to people who were different. When I was fifteen and sixteen I was already friends with boys who were gay, and I didn't even know what homosexuality was in those days.

I was eighteen when I met Alex at school, in St. Jerome. We immediately connected. At the time he had a boyfriend, Yves, whom he left after we began to go out. He talked to me about dance, the theatre, opera, things I also liked. It was wonderful. And Alex was the first person for whom I felt a sexual desire. Before, never.

At that time, when we met, I was highly emotional and dramatic, very high strung. Alex was calm. I was immediately attracted to his calm. He was attracted to my exuberance. From the point of view of personality, we were opposite. I brought to life his crazy side, and he evoked my calm side. We complimented each other. A perfect equilibrium.

Alex was a year older than me and began university in Montreal while I was still in my last year at CEGEP. I took dance classes in Montreal twice a week, and on those days we met at a metro station and came back to St. Jerome together. At one point he stopped coming home with me. When I asked him why, he said he had begun to see Yves again, who was now living in Montreal. And he thought he was in love. I went crazy. For a whole week I couldn't eat. I couldn't concentrate on anything. I thought he had left me forever. Then I thought, If it didn't last the first time, it's not going to last this time.

I went to Montreal and stayed with a friend of my mother's. Alex was staying in Montreal with his sister, and I kept walking up and down the street where he lived. One afternoon I decided to go upstairs. I rang the bell. His sister answered. Alex was working on a term paper for university. We started talking, and his sister went out to leave us alone. Within minutes we were making love on the floor. Alex told me things were not going well with Yves. I said, "Do you want to get back together?"

He said, "You know I also like guys."

"It doesn't matter."

"Let me think about it. I want to have relations with men, and even if you accept it, I don't know if I can. Give me some time."

One month later I was pregnant. There was no doubt in my mind: I had to get an abortion. I still wanted to go to university, I didn't want to be saddled with a child. I called Alex to tell him. He said, shouldn't you think about it? I said, "I've already thought about it. I'm only nineteen, I feel too much like a child myself to have a child. And I don't even know if we're going to be together."

He said, "I've made up my mind about us."

"I hope not because of the abortion."

"No, it's not working with Yves. I want us to get back together again."

I was starting university in a few months and we agreed to share an apartment in town. At university I took linguistics. I had taken ballet for years but didn't want to go into dance, I wasn't competitive enough. I thought to myself, I love words. I'll go into linguistics. But after a year I realized that studying linguistics is not literary. I studied and understood nothing.

In those days, I was always perfectly made up: lipstick, eye makeup, long polished nails, sophisticated clothes. I didn't look like a student. At university everyone dressed casually. And people didn't speak to me. People thought I was a snob. The first year I was totally alone. In some courses we had to work in groups, and I always ended up with the professor. No one was interested in working with me. No one talked to me, no one helped me. I realized it was because of the way I looked. But I wasn't about to change. And I didn't approach people, either. The second year I met a couple of gay guys and became friends with Eric. He told me he was intrigued that I didn't care what people thought of me and refused to conform.

Alex liked the way I dressed. He also liked people who were different. That's how he first noticed me. Every Saturday night we went dancing, and I was the star because of the way I dressed. I spent my spare time trying to invent new dresses, costumes to wear for Saturday night. Today I'm much more casual. But in those days I loved to dress in exotic, glamorous ways. I also used strange makeup. Striking colours. I never went out with as little makeup as I wear now, just lipstick with a bit of mascara.

Though Alex and I lived together, he also went out with guys. He even brought some of them home for supper and introduced them to me. I don't know if they knew Alex and I had a relationship. They might have thought we were good friends and just living together. Then one night he brought over Michel. I could see this person was different from the others. He wasn't just an affair. He was the kind of person Alex was really attracted to. The others weren't his type. It was just physical. Some were even street types, on the verge of delinquency. But Michel was very rooted, a successful actor. I could tell Alex was in love with him. He soon stopped sleeping with me, and we hardly saw each other. I started to get nervous. Three years after we had been living together, Alex said, "It's finished." And he moved into his own apartment.

I felt totally lost. I didn't know where to go, what to do. I couldn't make a decision. I didn't know whether to stay in the apartment or find something else. I put all my energy into school work.

Things went downhill with Michel, but Alex began to feel he was really homosexual, not bisexual, so even when his relationship with Michel ended he didn't want to move back with me. Five months later, the lease for the apartment ran out, and I still hadn't looked for another place. I asked Alex if I could move in with him. I said, "We'll sleep separately." He agreed, but it was hell for me. Each time he came in late or didn't come home, I couldn't sleep. I was still in love with him. Finally, we started to make love again. He said, "I've never seen anyone so persistent."

I said, "I love you. I will always love you, no matter what you do."

So we got back together again. He loved me, but he still had to face his homosexuality, and that confused him. He really was more attracted to men than to women. He didn't even look at women when we were on the street or in a club. At least I was enough for him. And his attraction to men didn't bother me. But when I saw him near another girl, I wanted to die. He could sleep with all the men in Montreal but not with another girl. And I know I'm the only girl he ever slept with. At least, in a way, he was faithful to me.

At one point, since Alex was going out with men, I was beginning to feel insecure and wondered if I could still be attractive to other men. I went to bars to pick up guys and slept with them. When I felt secure again I stopped. I told Alex after I did it.

He said, "If I can go outside of our relationship, so can you."

I said, "But I didn't go outside for sex. I went outside to see if I could still attract men."

After university, I tried to get work in linguistics but found nothing. I then took a course in accounting and got a job at Le Château doing inventory. Certainly not a place where I thought I'd end up. While doing linguistics, I had wanted to switch to dance. At the time, the university had just introduced courses in dance theory and practice. Since I had taken ballet for years, I auditioned for the course but wasn't accepted. Instead of trying to find another way of getting in, pushing, I sat down and cried. I didn't persevere. When it comes to a relationship, I persevere. But I haven't been able to develop a career. I don't have enough confidence. I get one rejection and I won't go back again.

Alex and I are very similar in not being able to fight for what we want. He got his degree in architecture but couldn't find work in his field, either. He ended up working for Unemployment Insurance as a civil servant, deciding who was eligible and who wasn't. Neither of us was really satisfied or happy with what we ended up doing. Alex had a talent for architecture but didn't have the confidence to follow through. I also could have done better, just judging by my grades. I finished university with a B+. I was conscientious, and I know I have the intelligence, but I can't channel that intelligence. I don't focus and stay with one project. Alex is the same way. Often he would start something and not finish. For instance, he should have confronted his homosexuality more than he did. He didn't take it to its logical end. He was always in a dilemma. He was with me but he was not fully satisfied. He needed men sexually. I think if I hadn't been so persevering he would have been fully homosexual.

We had a wonderful sexual relationship. I've never had anyone as good as him. But I wasn't enough for him. When he really wanted a man he became restless. He'd go out and not come back till the next morning. And I'd stay up waiting for him. I had wanted to leave him several times. But I loved him. For me, in every way, he was perfect.

In terms of taste, Alex and I liked exactly the same things. It was terrific. We were in total agreement about how to decorate the apartment. We never had any arguments over what dishes or furniture to buy, what colour to paint the rooms. We liked the same operas, the same singers, the same actors and actresses.

Alex's only fault was that he was a little impatient, otherwise he was very gentle, tender, loving, and generous. He cared about others and knew how to listen. And he was very good in the kitchen. He learned how to cook from his mother, and he took cooking classes at school. He did most of the cooking at home. He liked to sing. He read a lot. He liked going to the theatre. But he was a loner. He only had one or two friends. I was more gregarious.

Eight years after we met, we decided to get married, as a symbolic celebration of our love. There were thirty people at the wedding, and we had a wonderful party with all our friends. Almost all of them were gay since all my friends are gay.

With most gay men, the mother plays a large role in their life and the father is absent. I think I grew up with the same situation, that's why I get along so well with them. All my gay friends talk about their mothers, never about their fathers. I'm the same way. Alex was also very attached to his mother, and his father had ignored him.

When I go to a party, I will always end up talking to a gay guy, and we'll immediately click. I find them very creative, and there is no sexual tension. I'm uncomfortable with heterosexual men. I become very aggressive and defensive with them. I am always explaining and justifying myself. Always arguing. Always criticizing what they say. Even though I have problems with heterosexual men, it's men I'm attracted to. But I can easily be attracted to someone who is bisexual. I've even slept with homosexuals who have wanted to know what it was like to sleep with a girl. With gay men I feel perfectly comfortable. I can hug them, kiss them, be affectionate and know my actions will never be misinterpreted. I feel safe with them. I don't feel threatened.

Finding out that friends have AIDS is really difficult for me. When I hear of someone I know who has landed in hospital or who has died, it really affects me. A few months ago, I found out that a good friend of mine who was thirty-two and living in Paris died of AIDS. He had

had the virus for eight years and never wanted to talk about it. He tried to hide the fact that he even had AIDS. But he's hid all his life, not just the illness. After I got the news of his death, I was depressed for weeks. I thought, When will it be my turn? How long do I still have to live? Really, I'm thinking of myself. It's quite selfish. But also it brings back memories of when Alex was sick.

Before Alex became ill, we had lived a love story together. We had friends. We had Felix, our cat. We took trips, talked about having a child. We could discuss anything and everything. We went to ballets, operas, plays, concerts. This was my life, our life. I saw myself growing old like this. After Alex died, all the time I had devoted to loving him was now free. Plus I no longer had a future, and so the present took on a much greater significance.

When I was with Alex, I had never thought just about myself. I never thought about what I would like to do alone. It just never occurred to me. After he died, I only had myself to think about. I could do whatever I wanted. And I began taking piano lessons. When I was fifteen, I had taken piano for two years, so I wasn't starting from scratch, I could read music. Then I thought I would like to take voice lessons. My piano teacher suggested a wonderful singing teacher.

Learning how to sing properly is very physical. You have to breathe from the stomach. You have to be aware of your posture. After the first couple of lessons my sides actually hurt from practicing the movement of the breath. I had spasms in my stomach. The real pleasure of singing didn't come till a year after I started the lessons. At that point I began to have a little control over my voice, and I wasn't always thinking about the breathing and the body. And I could actually begin to pay attention to what I was singing.

Then my teacher suggested I join a choir to stabilize my voice. She introduced me to the leader of an amateur choir and he accepted me. I loved it immediately. I never sang in a group before. I had always sung alone or with Alex. Often we would learn the words of a song and sang together at home, just for ourselves. We even did *Carmen*. It was fun.

Choir practice was in a church, where it was so calm and peaceful. While others practiced their parts, I looked at the angels and the statues. I thought about life. Singing helped me to forget everything and took me beyond myself. When the choir sang together, there was no animosity. It was like we were one body, one harmony.

I also took a painting course at the university. During the three-hour course, I totally forgot about time, about problems. My sole focus was the painting. It was quite a challenge for me. It was a real test of my self-confidence. I was so pleased when I did a painting that I actually liked.

Then I joined an amateur theatre group, and last year I had a key role in the play we put on, where I had to act, sing, and dance. It was a wonderful experience, but I got shingles because of the stress and ended up in bed for three months.

At that point I realized I was doing too much. Piano on Monday, painting on Tuesday, voice lessons on Wednesday, choir practice on Thursday. Theatre classes. I had something on every night, and I never had any time for myself. Plus I saw my friends.

It became clear that I couldn't keep running from one thing to another. I enjoyed doing all the activities, and I'm glad I did them. I always thought, I better do all this before I become too ill to do anything. But now the time has come to stop doing. I need to learn to feel comfortable with myself, with my solitude. This time the pain of the shingles was much worse than the last time, when Alex landed in hospital. I needed to listen to my body, and it was an effort. I always want to do more than I can. I push myself. Even for my friends I do more than I need to. I put myself out. I now need to learn to be. I need to deal with death and be ready for it. I don't know how much more time I have left.

After I had the attack of shingles, I began to leave days open. I had to know there was time when I didn't have anything to do. And soon I will have nothing at all to do but stay in bed. Before, I always scheduled myself. I had something to do all hours of the day, every day of the week. Not now. And it doesn't even bother me. A year ago, I would have felt terrible saying no when someone asked me to do something. Now I can do it. It's taken some work. I always had a problem saying no. I'm just starting to learn to do it. "No, I'm too tired." Or, "No, I have other things to do." Or simply, "No, I don't feel like it." It's important to choose what you give energy to. Before I didn't value energy. Now I need to conserve my energy. I can't waste it. Now, instead of being with friends, I do a lot of things alone. Wanting to be alone is recent.

When I wake up in the morning and feel good, I do what I can during the day. If I don't feel well, I stay in bed. I try to listen to myself. I'm learning that the most important person in this life is me. I think of others, and I like others, but I have to first please myself. I have to feel good with myself before feeling good with others. If I'm in a situation I don't like, I'm going to be very uncomfortable, and it can make me sick. I'm discovering and appreciating the subtleties of life more and more, and I see how they affect me.

When I'm calm I can sense people. But I pick up people's feelings too much. I'm trying to work on maintaining a distance when someone is talking to me. The other day a friend's dog disappeared. I spent hours thinking about his dog, hoping he'll be found soon. I don't need to take on people's worries. I wish I wouldn't do that. Also, sometimes I waste a lot of time thinking about what happened yesterday, and why didn't this happen instead of that. I replay events. I analyze them. After a while I realize this is stupid. What happened yesterday is finished. But I'm so used to rethinking events that I have a hard time to bring myself into the present.

Not only do I need to pay attention to myself when I'm alone, I also need to watch myself when I'm with others. I try not to be pulled into negative energies. I listen to people talk about their problems, like car problems, and I think, If you have a problem, solve it, why talk about it for hours on end? I feel life is a piece of theatre, a bit of a farce. People worry over nothing. I try to stay clear of a discussion about problems, complaints. Some people complain about all sorts of little things, like there are not enough parking places, the waiter at the restaurant is too slow, the cashier is rude. I listen to them and think, Why does it matter that it takes you fifteen minutes to find a parking place? It's not so important.

When I witness a conflict between people I no longer interfere.

Before, I would jump in, take sides, defend a position. Not now. When people tell me things, I try to see the positive side of whatever they're saying.

I'm also discovering that it's so much better to listen. Usually, while someone is telling us something, we're thinking of our response instead of listening. It's always I, I, I. Before, I don't think I really listened to people. I was more concerned about what I had to say. Now I try to talk less and less about myself. Before, I easily talked about myself, too easily, without thinking. It never bothered me. Now I become uncomfortable when I talk too much about myself. When I tell people very intimate things, I feel nude. This happens to me more and more often, and I don't like it. It's almost like I'm becoming aware of my feelings and I'm listening to them. When you're busy doing, you don't stop to think how you're feeling. Now, my feelings are becoming more and more important.

After spending too much time with people, I need fresh air. Particularly because recently I've noticed how often conversations are steeped in banality. Sometimes people talk about the intimate parts of their lives so freely that it makes what they're saying seem trite. I listen to people talk about themselves so easily and indiscriminately, and I think, My God, that's what I used to do. Before, I spoke too much. It's not necessary for everyone to know everything. These days I don't want people to know too much about me. I feel very private.

One thing that really bothers me is when I'm in the hospital waiting room and everyone is talking about their illnesses. That's all they talk about. Inevitably someone will turn to me to ask what I have. The last time I said, "I don't want to talk about it."

And this woman said, "But it's good to talk about it."

I said, "I talk about it with people I know. I don't want to talk about it with strangers."

She was very offended.

This summer, I had another outbreak of shingles. I was in such pain I was sure I was going to die. And I felt very lonely. I wanted people to look after me, but my friends weren't there. I would have liked them to come and visit me more. Very few came. Even the ones who did come only came once. It's hard to say anything to them because I'm proud. Of course, I have a problem asking for help. I'm always afraid of wasting people's time, of imposing myself. Also, I'm afraid people will say no.

To call someone and ask them to come over and look at my stereo is easier than to ask them to come over because I need someone with me or I need to talk. I'm so afraid the person will say, Yes, I'll come over, but they do it out of obligation, not necessarily because they want to. It's important for me to know that people are doing something for me because they really want to. One friend has said, "When you ask me for something, I'm afraid to say no because you're so disappointed, and then I feel so guilty."

I said, "Well, I express my emotions. If I ask you for something and you say no, I can't casually just say, that's all right. I understand you can't do it, but I'm disappointed. I don't expect you to drop everything and just do what I ask. But I'm not going to say I don't mind if you can't come when I would have liked you to come."

When I'm feeling fine, everyone calls. When things are not going well, no one is there. Eric, my best friend, keeps his distance when I'm sick. This last time, I was in bed for a month and heard nothing from him for a week. A friend of his told me Eric is afraid when I'm sick. But when I'm sick, I need people I like around me. I was very upset that he didn't call. When I was feeling better, I called him. I said, "I need you when I'm not feeling well. When you don't call me I think you've had enough of my illness. You're getting fed up with me."

He said, "I'm just afraid. I prefer not to call you than to get bad news."

I said, "You're thinking of yourself, not me."

He said, "It's true, you're right." He cried. "Your illness really affects me. I think about it every day. I even went to see a psychologist. I can't imagine you sick."

I said, "I understand, but I need to hear from you. When I'm sick, talking to you only once a week is not enough." It was hard for me to tell him that.

When things aren't going well, I want people to be able to sense what I'm going through. I don't want to have to tell them. If I had a friend who I knew had AIDS, I would do more for him than what my friends do for me. If Eric were sick, I would set aside my Saturdays for him. I would take him for walks. I would do his shopping for him. And if I knew he didn't have much money, I would pay for his groceries, if I could afford it.

My friends are so certain that, because I'm always positive and usually in a good mood, I'm self-sufficient. They see me as someone full of energy, and even when I complain I do it with humour. They think I'm strong. But being strong mentally doesn't mean I'm also strong physically. And it doesn't eliminate my need for them emotionally. My friends are so used to me always taking the initiative that they don't realize I need more from them now than before. They keep thinking everything will be fine. They don't realize these are the last months that we're going to share together. It's fragile. I really feel I don't have much time left. Very often I feel I'm already in another world.

I'd like to talk about my coming end with friends and family. Unfortunately, to date, they haven't wanted to talk about it. When I begin to talk about death, they say, "Don't think about that." But I need to talk. That's a dilemma for me. I think if people would be willing to listen they would benefit from my dying, my death. I could help them to live a richer life. My experience of this illness could help others.

Precisely because I am not free to talk about death, I feel a certain anxiety. I'm not afraid of death, but I feel bad for my friends. I see myself in the hospital with my mouth open, pale, hardly enough energy to talk, and people crying around me. I don't want people to be hurt because of me. I don't want my illness to be painful for them. When the time comes for me to die, I want people to talk to me about life. I want them to be happy around me. I want to have some humour around my death as well as a few very intense moments. Also, I would like to talk to certain people, as Alex did.

I can accept death, but I don't want to suffer. Suffering serves no purpose. I have no patience for suffering. When I decide it's time to go, I'll stop taking my pills, and it'll happen quickly. I don't think I'll linger too long. I will simply let myself go. Though I think I will have to be pretty strong in order to be able to do that. But I don't think of death as a finality. There is something beyond.

It'll be interesting to see what's on the other side. There will be souls without any barriers between them. All will be one. I know that love surrounds us, and I sometimes feel it here on earth. These days I see a lot of white and mauve light. Sometimes I'm walking on the street, my feet are on the ground, but I feel beyond everything that's around me, detached from it, and it's very pleasant. I think, If this is what's going to happen, it'll be beautiful.

In the past couple of weeks, I've been feeling very ill and need to sleep more and need more time to myself. I'm trying to find and develop an inner peace before I leave. Now I can tune into my own calm and hold it, but that's been very recent. I sometimes try to think of the light I saw when Alex was dying. It calms me. I think Alex will come and help me die. Then he'll let me do the rest of the journey on my own. Later we'll meet up again.

I do feel lighter these days. Easier. Recently I definitely feel I live in two realities. The other day I felt my soul next to my body. I was walking on the street and felt as if someone was beside me all the time. I wondered if it was Alex.

At night I sometimes feel my soul moving around me like loose clothing. I see myself really large. I fill the room. The walls ripple and move farther and farther away. I feel as if I've lost touch with everything around me. But things seem very real in that state. More real than reality. And I get answers to my questions. But it's hard to stay with it. It's like vertigo.

From time to time I've had this same feeling during the day as well. I become hyperconscious of everything. My body feels larger than it is, and I don't want to touch anyone. When someone just brushes against me, it feels like an electric shock. Then at times I feel outside of my body, detached, and watch myself eating or talking.

When I'm at peace, I can feel my soul fully in place around me and I feel a tremendous love for people. I feel my body opening, and

I want to touch people more than usual. I want them to touch me. There's this surge of love within, and I want to embrace everyone. I feel like putting my arms around the whole world. That's the feeling I want to have when I die.

When Alex died I felt such peace around him that it entered me. And then I lost it. Recently I have become infused with his peace again. Now I can feel it almost the way I felt it when he died. I take that as a sign that it's time. And I'm ready.

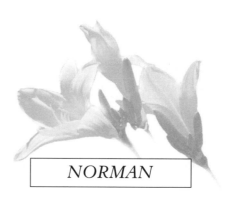

NORMAN

A doctor at a palliative care unit gave me Norman's name, saying, "I think he would be happy to talk. He has not yet faced his death, but perhaps in speaking with you he will."

Norman, seventy-six, was dying of lung cancer. He had a private room on the palliative care unit. He was happy for the opportunity to talk. He had big, bright blue eyes that were on the alert, curious, welcoming whatever presented itself. When I walked into his room to introduce myself, he very graciously extended his hand and welcomed me with a big smile that lit up his face. He was lean, with thinning grey hair, and his manner was always gentlemanly.

As he told his story, there was almost a childish glee in his voice when relating pleasant memories. But that glee could easily turn to sadness, tears, or anger when he moved to other episodes. He shifted easily between different emotions, willing to feel their full extent. He had no reason to suppress any feelings with me, something I think he must have done most of his life, and he freely let the full force of his emotions cascade over him. He cried readily when he talked about sad memories, and when I apologized for having asked questions that evoked tears, he simply said, "That's all right, the tears have to come. It's good."

During our third interview, when I asked him how he felt about

the end, he got very angry and refused to talk. I quickly had to backtrack.
At the next interview, I broached the subject from another angle. This
time he was more open.

I've been in hospital since January. Three months. It gets boring
sometimes. I count the spots on the wall. I find all kinds of things to
count. And I keep thinking about leaving. But I have no idea when
I'll have the strength. It'll be quite a while. I'm sleeping more and
more, getting weaker and weaker. It's very frustrating. I can't move
without a person on each side of me. How on earth am I going to get
out of here this way? I have no energy to even talk to people anymore. My sister comes in to visit every day, and last Tuesday I asked
her to only come every second day. That's plenty. I want to see fewer
and fewer people. I want to sleep. Maybe if I get a good sleep I'll feel
better. Maybe the cancer in my lungs will not act up so much. There
was a time when I lived with it and it didn't bother me. I was just fine.

The tumour was diagnosed about a year ago, when I was admitted
to hospital for tests. Then I found out it was cancer and felt terrible.
Emotionally I felt cut off from everything. Life suddenly comes to a
dead stop when you realize what's happening. But I must say I had
plenty of warning. I mean, for anyone in my position, being a heavy
smoker, it was bound to occur. As soon as the doctor mentioned tests
and the hospital, I knew that was the end of my smoking. But, as a
life-long smoker, I wasn't going to just give in. I was scheming, trying
to find different ways of accomplishing my ends. While in hospital,
I kept saying, I want to go to the bathroom, but you can only play that
so often.

After the tests, when I got out of the hospital, I continued to smoke.
My condition grew worse and worse. I was living alone, a bachelor,
and eventually I could no longer cook for myself or go to the bathroom. I couldn't manoeuvre anymore. I was so weak. The funny part
was, I couldn't eat anything, either. You'd think you would be able to
help yourself by eating to fight off the fatigue, but I just couldn't. My
friends had been taking care of me for some time. They straightened

out my apartment and did all the necessary things. Then came a crisis where I was coughing, having problems breathing, and the boys called the ambulance. While waiting for it to arrive, I was nervous because I'm not a person who goes to the hospital very often. In my seventy-six years, this was to be my third time in. It felt like I was waiting to go on a trip I didn't want to take. There was all the anticipation, but it wasn't very enjoyable. I knew this was serious. I had no choice about this trip. Before the ambulance arrived, I lit up a cigarette, then put the package down, and that was it. No more cigarettes. Getting sick might have been the best thing that happened to me. How else was I going to stop smoking?

It was only after I was in hospital for a while that I began to eat. And I started to recover. I say recover because I feel much better than when I came in here. Now I eat three meals a day instead of none. That makes a big difference. I sit up in a nice easy chair, have my dinner, and I stay there for about an hour. It gives me something to look forward to, and it gives me some exercise. Then I get back into bed again.

The doctor did say I could arrange to have a smoke. There is a little cubbyhole in the basement for smokers. For staff and patients. But I didn't like the atmosphere. There was no air, and it was too hard to get there with a wheelchair. It was too far. I was in no condition to go there alone. And I wasn't going to ask a nurse to wheel me down.

It's going to take so long to get in shape. Just thinking about it is discouraging. I would like to regain my strength to walk around again. But what would that give me? Maybe a few more years? I could go out with the boys again. Or it would give me nothing.

I'm sad when I think of the way it used to be. I wasn't much for going out and having a hell of a time, as they say. I was more a homebody. I wasn't running around all over. I was just an ordinary guy, enjoying myself and enjoying my friends. Life was great. I had a nice TV. I used to cook for myself, although I hated cooking. Hated it. I liked to do a lot of reading, newspapers and historical books. I loved history, even recent history. The war. Books are rather expensive, so I used to buy them from the Book-of-the-Month Club. I had to give it up just before I came in here. Couldn't keep up anymore, nor could I concentrate on reading. I can't concentrate on much now. Can barely get through some of my meals these days.

I don't know why I feel so weak. Can't do anything anymore. Can barely pick up a knife and fork. The nurses have to give me a bath, and some of them are rough. There are only two nurses I allow to give me a bath, my two favourites, Annie and Heather. The others I don't want to see anymore.

It's even hard to see my friends, and they're wonderful. They come in to visit regularly and do everything for me. Audrey, who is sixty and the mother of one of my young friends, has taken a liking to me. She's become a good friend. She lives just across the street, so she comes in with the newspaper every morning on her way to work. Five days a week. She stands at the foot of the bed and touches my leg so I can feel she's there. She comes in every evening, too. We yak. She does the little laundry I have and buys me the personal stuff I need. Sometimes we buy a couple of loto tickets together. This past week I won $10. I also let her do my banking.

I didn't know what to think of it at first, someone who would do all that for you. How am I going to show my appreciation? I'm on my back. I can't do nothing. "Stay on your damn back," she says. "When you get better, we'll go out."

We talked about going to the Rib'N Reef for some good roast beef when I get out. I like roast beef, nice and thick and juicy. Oh man, just the thought. We talk about that.

Audrey has two sons. I'm friends with the older one, Steve. He's married now. Has a family and a good job with Air Canada. He's exceptional. He comes down here Tuesdays and Thursdays to make sure I have everything I need. He shaves me. Helps me with my meals. Helps me to sit up. I'm very lucky.

My friends, the boys, are young, all in their late twenties. They call me up nearly every day. If I need anything, they're down here like a shot. "What is it? What can we do?" They generally know because as soon as they come in that door they see what's happening and take care of me.

❧

You'd be surprised how I met such young people at my late age. And they're just out of this world. I met Steve on Christmas Day, eleven years ago, three months after I retired. I was going home from Murray's Restaurant, and there was a terrible ice storm. Decided to take a taxi home, even though I lived only a few blocks away. After I got out of the car and as I closed the door, I did an awful slip. My foot got caught in something, and I twisted the whole thing. Steve and his friends happened to be by and saw me sprawled on the ground. They offered to help me into my apartment. It was very kind. Once I was in, I felt all right and told them I didn't need any more help. What a mistake that was! I walked on a bad leg for three or four days. It became more and more painful till I finally had to see a doctor, who sent me to be X-rayed. He immediately saw something was wrong. It seems I had broken my foot after I got out of that taxi. The doctor immediately put me in hospital and scheduled an operation. They had to amputate my left leg. That time I stayed in hospital for well over a month.

After the operation, I used crutches to get around. I didn't want any other means of transport, like a wheelchair. The crutches were enough. A few days after I was discharged from hospital, I was trying to walk about on the street. I had to stop for a rest by a street light. Steve happened to be around there at the time and spotted me. He came running over, wanting to know what had happened and did I want any help. From then on, he took me under his wing, coming to see me every day to see if I needed anything. He lived nearby, just a block away. Then I met Tim and Mike, friends of Steve. I have three of them. The three musketeers. At the time I was sixty-four and they were eighteen or nineteen. We've been friends ever since, even though I'm old enough to be their father or even grandfather.

When I met the boys, they were single and just starting university. They more or less reached adulthood in my place. They had their drinks there. The four of us sometimes went out to supper together. Then we'd come back to my apartment, put on the TV, and watch our special programs, especially hockey. We liked arguing about the scores.

It was a nice atmosphere. Used to be two or three of us all the time. It was good.

Then they met their girlfriends. One of the first things they did was to bring the girlfriends over to introduce them to me. I guess I had to get their approval. They'd come in to see who this old guy was. I got along with the three girls perfectly. It was wonderful. Then both the boys and girls came to visit me in the apartment. The girls didn't come as often. They had their own get-togethers and we had ours. Not uproarious, just a few beers and discussions. Very nice, wonderful.

Then they got married and I went to their weddings. I enjoyed every minute of it. Every minute. Then Tim's little girl came along. Now they all live in the West Island, have nice homes, good jobs. It's very refreshing that I don't have to worry about whether they have a job or not. All three of them have good, stable jobs. I can be proud. They're my family now. I'm very happy with them. Gotta be happy, can't be sad all the time.

As a whole, I have no profound regrets. I have regrets, but I figure as long as I did my best with everyone I met, that was good enough. I figure I did my share. Maybe not my total share, but part of my share. Maybe it's not good enough. Life takes twists and turns. Lots of places I would have still loved to go but you can't go everywhere, so you're satisfied. Besides, I was always a homebody.

Since I retired at sixty-three, till I got sick a year ago, these last thirteen years have been the happiest I've had. I was financially independent. I was living on my pension, so I wasn't wanting for cash. I was living a life of leisure. Life was rather pleasant and everything was so handy. I lived on Sherbrooke Street West, near here, in a nice apartment that I enjoyed very much. I had moved into the building after I retired. I think I was very accepted and felt good living there. There were stores all around, a bank nearby, restaurants. Was able to get around without any trouble. It was just wonderful. Except for the operation on my leg, I must say I think these were the happiest years. Of course, I would never have met the boys if not for the accident and the leg. Things have a funny way of turning out.

Before retirement, I worked at CN for twenty-seven years. The last twelve years I did the four to twelve shift. Before that I sometimes did the day shift or the midnight shift. I hated that one. CN ran the business of air express for Air Canada. I enjoyed most of the work, though some parts I hated, like the shipment of life-saving medicine, and we had a lot of that. It's very nerve-wracking when you have someone depending on you whether they live or die. Managing orders, seeing that things get done takes a tremendous amount of time and a large staff. And there's never enough time or enough people. Naturally, that creates problems. But customers never seem to understand that. It spoils your fun completely.

From the sublime to the ridiculous, I also hated the shipping of dogs and cats. Our policy was to give only an approximate flight. We could never guarantee a flight because anything could happen between the depot and the plane. But the customers always wanted to know exactly when their pets were going to arrive. Used to make me sick. Factories also depended on parts that needed to arrive by a certain time, usually the sooner the better. It was quite a pressure job. There were times when I was very happy to leave at the end of my shift. I liked to close the door behind me and say, "Thank God for another night!"

But I did enjoy the bookkeeping and seeing the increase in user-ship. It was a terrific business. Now Purolator and Loomis are making a fortune, and Air Canada is falling behind. Makes me mad. I think they should be the first because they have the equipment, the aircraft, the pilots, the crew. They should be making a pile of money and they're not. You have to ask yourself a few questions. But there was not much I could do. You're only a small guy in a big pond.

If everybody had done their job properly, things would have been different. Things would have gotten done. But people can get into silly arguments with each other over nothing. I've tried to change that, the way people act toward one another. But you can't help that. There is no use trying. It never worked. If you had a problem or if you were really sick, most of them wouldn't lift a finger to help. They'd just ignore you. It happened to me once. I had a very bad flu. I couldn't shave or do anything, and it was very hard to get someone to replace me. Some of them could have very well done it but chose not to. It hurts, things like that. Nothing much you can do about it, and once it's done, it's done. You can't undo it. I'll get over it. You have to get over it if you want to continue.

I didn't have close friends. I didn't talk to anyone. I was what you would call a loner, I guess. I did have ordinary acquaintances. I might have had supper with them once in a while, but I was not very close to them. Once, years ago, there was someone I liked very much. A very nice guy.

One day at work a fellow came in desperately needing a job. He was down and out, on his last legs. I thought, I'll take a chance. I couldn't give him the job myself, but other people could. I introduced him to the right contacts, gave him the nod. The company was looking for permanent people at the time. That was the only thing he let me down on, he didn't stay. There was nothing I could do. Can't hold a man against his will. He stayed about seven or eight months. We became real buddies.

He was very good-hearted, that's what I liked about him. Very good-hearted. If he saw someone down and out he wouldn't pass him by. He would always stop and give him something. There aren't many people who care about others and their troubles and he'd go back and give the person whatever he had to make sure he could get a meal. I used to like that. I did a lot of that myself. It seemed natural to help people. If you're doing all right, doesn't mean everyone else is. You have to share with somebody. I used to help them out. I was glad to do it. You don't always want something back. You just do it because you want to do it. Ray was the same way.

Although he cared for people, he had a sort of a carefree attitude. He gave you that carefree feeling — I got nothing to worry about, I'm as free as a bird. I liked that. He didn't take anything too seriously, he'd laugh things off, joke about things. I guess maybe I took life too seriously. Sometimes I took myself too seriously. I don't think I ever felt carefree. I thought he'd settle down. I thought everything was going all right for a while, but it wasn't.

He was a wanderer, just couldn't stop wandering. He'd stop for a while, be as happy as anything, then he'd get the wanderlust. Poor guy. I used to feel so sorry for him. When you keep wandering around like that, you have to come to rest somewhere. Of course, that was my stupidity. I figured you have to settle down, set up home, set up shop like I should have done.

One Sunday poor Ray just disappeared. He didn't let me know he was planning to leave, that was the queerest thing. One day he was here and the next day he was gone. He didn't give me a clue. He doesn't warn you or anything. That's the way he is, just goes. I was very hurt. And I missed him, his carefree ways, his attitude toward everything. But all good things come to an end. Just one of those things. It's always been that way.

Ray, God knows where he is now. I hope he's doing all right. I still think about him sometimes. I still miss him.

Then a few years later I lost my stepmother. I felt very lonely after that. She was the closest person to me. We had lived together from the time my father died, when I was seventeen, till the day she went.

I loved her. She was so good, very kind. She did housekeeping and cooking for me. She liked to surprise me, cook different foods I enjoyed. She would hide the vegetables or the meat so I wouldn't see them and guess we were going to have a special treat. It's these little things that make up everything. She'd do it so beautifully. She knew I loved strawberry shortcake, and when that time came around, I knew I was going to get some, but I didn't know when. She used to fool me sometimes, had me believe she wasn't going to make it one year, and then, suddenly, there was a nice big chunk of strawberry shortcake. Boy, it was good. She made it all herself, the cake, whipped the cream, hand-picked the strawberries from the store. Sometimes you get spoiled. I didn't do anything special to deserve it. Yes, I supported her, but after all, she was my stepmother. I felt it was my responsibility to see she had what she wanted and needed, and I used to try to provide that as best I could.

℘

She began to get sick when I was in my late forties. She was old and not very well. Even then she was so considerate. She'd say, "Never mind I'll be all right."

And I knew she was going to suffer. She had a bad rheumatic condition and she went blind a few years before she died. It was very hard for her. We arranged things in the house so she wouldn't hurt herself. Then she'd wait for me to get home to do the necessary cooking. I'd stand beside her to make sure she didn't touch the hot stove accidentally. At the end I did the cooking for the two of us. I was quite happy taking care of her. After all, she had taken care of me for quite a while, so why shouldn't I take care of her?

She passed away in hospital at the age of seventy-eight. I was with her when she died on Christmas Day, two o'clock. That made it very hard. I felt terrible. Terrible. But you had to get over it. She was so good. Those were hard days. I missed her so much. She had a beautiful personality and I inherited it, so there. You can't take that away from me. I'd do the same again for her.

As time went on, after my stepmother died, I often thought about changing jobs, but one was as bad as the other. I didn't try to find another job very hard, not hard enough. You get yourself in a groove and you're sort of stuck in it. And when you're getting old, it's pretty hard. For a while I was happy at CN. But then the work I once liked I started to hate. Not much you can do about that. I became more and more nervous. The nervousness just gradually came on sometime after my stepmother died. I guess these things start little by little. It came like anything else, I guess. After a while I felt like a bundle of nerves. Irritable. For no reason at all, you can be very irritable with a customer or with your co-workers. Patience wasn't even in my vocabulary. Patience was just a word. When I got home from work in the evenings, I was very tired. I had problems sleeping. It was no good.

No one said anything at work except my bosses. They told me to have the problem attended to. I went to see the doctor because I could feel this wasn't natural. The doctor wanted to know a bit of history. I told him about the parts that were bothering me at work, about the dogs and cats and the damn medicine. All that stuff. The incessant ringing of the phones, phones, phones. Everything ringing at once.

One thing leads to another. After a while I just blew a gasket. I had a nervous breakdown. Don't ask me why. I couldn't stand anything. I grew very sensitive. Too sensitive. Things that used to be routine got to be a big mess, a big to-do. It was impossible. The doctor told me I better make up my mind whether I wanted to stay there or leave. I decided to take my pension. I had that choice. I was lucky to blow when I could retire.

I retired in the fall and felt great. Who wouldn't? I was relaxed for the first time in I can't remember how many years. If I could have afforded it, I would have done it ten years earlier. But everything straightens out. You forgive and forget. Or that's the way it's supposed to be. What's gone is gone, and what's to come is to come. Not much you can do about things that are said and done.

Sometimes my life seemed a little out of whack, but it always straightened itself out, came back to the old pendulum, back to normal again. You tolerate what you can tolerate. I'm used to it now, had to get used to it early in life.

When I was only two years old and my sister was about ten, my mother died. After her death, my sister was adopted by a rich aunt, my father's sister, who had no children of her own. She was very lucky. She had a good life. We'd see one another from time to time. Not that often. My sister never talked to me about our mother, and we weren't allowed to see my mother's parents. My father's sister stopped us from seeing them, and she tolerated no talk of my mother.

My father never mentioned my mother, either. He was a harsh and sometimes cruel man. He'd beat you up for the smallest thing. That's where my stepmother came in, she'd interfere to make sure I didn't get hurt. My stepmother cared for me. She was very good. I always liked her. She'd come in to protect me when he was beating me too hard. He didn't beat me that often, maybe once a month. But when you got a beating, you remembered it. It hurt. In later years I was very happy my sister was independent of any goings-on, happy that she didn't have to go through anything. These beatings hurt both inside and out. Don't know which was worse. I didn't think I deserved all of them, but he did, and that's what counted the most. I'm still here, anyway.

I wasn't close to my father. He wasn't the kind of person you take to very easily. I think he found it very hard to show any affection whatsoever to his kids. So he just ignored them. You were there but you weren't there.

My father was a civil servant, and he wasn't even around that long. In spite of everything, I would have liked him to be around longer. When I was seventeen, he had a stroke and within a week was a goner. I wouldn't have thought he'd go so quickly. I thought he was stronger.

I spent a year alone with my stepmother and at eighteen enlisted for the war. Before being shipped out, I was first sent to Calgary for six months to take a wireless radio course. That's when I met Marge, the only girl I ever loved. She was so wonderful. She could make you laugh. She wasn't a beautiful girl. I'm not going to say, like a hundred million others, she was a beautiful girl. No, she wasn't. But she was a down-to-earth girl and so smart. Such a beautiful personality. When we raced to the tree in her back yard, she loved to beat me, and we'd laugh about it. She had a wonderful sense of humour, always playing tricks on me, like hiding stuff you thought you had. You were looking for it, couldn't find it, and you swore you had it. Then she'd turn up with it. I was in constant laughter over her tricks.

We wouldn't get married before I went to war. We didn't believe in that spur-of-the moment thing. We wanted to make sure. I'm one of those, I've got to be sure. Though we were practically engaged before I left.

After the wireless radio course, I was sent to a gunnery school in Ontario, near Guelph, where we were taught to take direct aim and shoot. During the course in Calgary, I had made a lot of friends. When I was transferred, I hoped some of them would also be sent there. And some were. I was happy about that. Some of the old diehards came with me. A month later, we were shipped overseas. During the war, I didn't see Marge for a long time. Five years. We used to correspond.

I was all over England, Scotland, Wales. Then I participated in the invasion of North Africa. We operated out of Gibraltar, which was our base.

The war was quite an adventure, but it didn't give me anything except grief. When somebody in the crew died, sometimes the others used to speak very lightly of it. I couldn't take anybody being frivolous about people dying. I just walked away. I couldn't stand when someone joked about death. Every day it's going on. You see people dying around you. You're shooting at people. Still, I didn't go for it. I used to get very angry. Don't talk to me in a silly way about death. When your friends leave for battle, you say goodbye to them in your own way, and then they don't come back. They're missing. It affects you. You can't help it. You can't forget it. That part is terrible. We had to win the war, but it was very hard to take, very hard. But I got through it, I guess.

As soon as the war was over I went out to Calgary to see Marge. I had all kinds of schemes to see her. You had to scheme because you had to have a good reason to get the travel permits to go from Montreal to Calgary. I stayed in Calgary a couple of months. It was wonderful, just like a honeymoon. She lived with her mother and father, and they were members of the United Church, very strict. No smoking, no dancing, and no this and no that. Kids wouldn't tolerate it today. It used to drive me crazy. She felt the same way but was scared to disobey her parents. She did disobey them, but we had to sneak around. Her parents knew who she was out with, so they weren't worried. They liked me.

We used to go to the big hotel in Calgary, where they had nice dances. There were no bars in those days. And both Marge and I liked rye and ginger ale. You could buy a bottle at the liquor store, but you weren't allowed to show it. We took the liquor in a bag to the hotel, where Marge and I made sure we sat near a big plant, and we'd hide the bottle in the planter. We had fun with that. Sometimes four of us went together and shared a bottle.

When I left Calgary, we had a loose agreement. We wanted to meet one another again, see one another again. We knew we had a big block between us on this religion thing. I was Roman Catholic and she was from the United Church, and in those days that was a big problem for me. Marge wasn't religious, but her parents were. I wanted her to become a Catholic. Both my mother and father had been Catholic, and I wanted to uphold the tradition. I felt it was my responsibility. In those days it did make a difference to your whole family and all your friends.

In hindsight, now, I would marry her even if she wouldn't become a Roman Catholic, but then I couldn't. Just the circumstances. My stepmother was a practicing Protestant. That's what made it so difficult. I was trying to hold up my end. I nearly weakened. What could I do? At the time I wasn't really a practicing Catholic, but I had to argue if I wanted to get married. We used to argue pro and con. Marge didn't like parts of the Catholic religion, like the compulsory confession.

Three months after I left Calgary, she came to meet me in Toronto for the last time to see if we could work it out. She stayed for two months. I asked her in a million ways to become a Catholic. She wouldn't. We enjoyed everything else till it came to that damn subject. She was still very good, even in the misunderstandings. Wonderful. After two months I put her on the train, said goodbye, and that was the last I saw of her. We agreed not to see each other till we could resolve this religion question.

We kept in touch for a long time, but then we couldn't stand it any longer, so we thought the best thing for the both of us was to break the relationship and see if we could do better elsewhere. Neither one of us was allowed to contact the other. We were going to let each other be happy with whoever we met next. I felt terrible. Even today I feel so terrible, not knowing what happened to her, not knowing anything.

I don't like to talk about it. It's too hard even at this late age. I have kept it to myself all these years, so I guess I can do it for a few more.

My stepmother knew about Marge. She thought I was a bit nuts. I think she thought I should have married her but never said as much. She said, "It's for you to settle your own life." She would have approved of whatever I had done. It was a sad state of affairs. I didn't want to give in, and she didn't want to give in. I loved her and she loved me. It was a stupid way to break up. A stupid reason.

If I could do it over again, I would definitely marry her. And the hell with the opinion of others. I regret not having married her. Nearly every day of my life I think of it. I should have given in. Why did I have to be the strong one? She was so wonderful. So stupid. It'll never be undone.

What's gone is gone. It doesn't do either me or her any good thinking about it now. Isn't that terrible? Why am I doing this? Why bring it all up now? Should keep my emotions under control. It hurts all right. I never like to think of it anymore. There are things that hurt, but you don't want to say anything. I'm too old to impress anybody now. There are a few years I'd love to relive.

It hurts, bringing up the very basics of your life. It hurts, but like all the hurts, it'll dull up a bit. I was wrong. I should have compromised. I don't know how to compromise, but there should have been a compromise. It was so stupid. There is nothing I can do about it now, and I'll never, never forgive myself. I missed a whole life, a family, a home. I'll never forgive myself for that. There should always be a little give here and a little give there. It should have been possible. All the good times we could have had.

Things could have been so different, and it didn't turn out. Had I not joined up and gone to war, maybe we would have gotten married. But then, if I had not joined up, I wouldn't have met her. Who knows? It was a very sad time.

When I came back from the war I was altogether different. You don't have your usual gang around you. But you had to get used to it. I got used to it. I remained friends with some of them, but it's hard to get across country. You have to have the money to travel around. I had a hard time, I must admit. After the war, I found it lonesome at first. I was a lot more serious, withdrawn from everything for a while. I was sort of a humourless creature when I came back. I couldn't see the humour in things anymore. I couldn't laugh anymore. But I got over that, thank God. But at the time I thought I would never do it. It took me a good year to get over it. I used to get very depressed. Very depressed. I think it had a lot to do with me not getting married.

Marge was such a wonderful girl, not that she had all the beauty, but that personality, God. She had such a way of asking you to do something, you'd fall on your face to do it. The little things mean a lot. Oh, well. You can't go around with a chip on your shoulder. You have to take life as it comes. It's strange. I don't think I had a chip on my shoulder. I could have had one.

I haven't had an uproarious life by any means, but then I never really wanted that. I don't like sudden uproars. I like it nice and quiet, like don't-rock-the-boat type of thing. My life has been all right, I guess, but if I had it to do over again, Jesus, would it ever be different.

There have been very few outstanding things in my life. I'd have to search. The only thing I can think of is my friends, Steve and the boys. They have made me very happy. I'm very proud of them. Almost like having my own sons. I often think of that. Would be nice if they had plenty of kids running around. I like kids. I love kids. They bring life to a gathering. Tim's daughter was a year old in July, and they're expecting another one soon. I saw the little girl just the other day. Before I ended up in hospital, I went to visit them as often as I could. In this last stretch of my life, I've acquired a family. One of them is bound to call me up tonight to see how I'm doing, what I'm having for supper. But the boys don't replace Marge. No one could ever replace Marge.

I'm making a fool of myself. You're not supposed to show emotion and here I am crying my eyes out. Things come up in your mind that have been dormant for years, and it comes to the surface and makes you very emotional. These things are important to me, very important.

In your own small way you enjoy talking about it. It brings up memories. It stirs up fires that haven't been stirred for years that maybe need stirring. I would have liked two nice girls and two sons. I would have liked that very much. Two of each. Would have been so wonderful, would have made my whole life. Instead you end up with nothing. I really feel I ended up with nothing. Nothing to show for my life, no kids coming in calling me Daddy.

My sister, she comes down every second day. She's older and in much better health than I am. She's not married, either. We're both old bachelors. Stupid thing to run in the family. Had she wanted to get married, she could have. If there was anything in the past, if she ever loved anybody, I don't know. She never spoke about it. She doesn't seem to have any regrets. She's quite religious now.

It's only lately that I believe in Catholicism, and it's for my sister's sake, who is a strong Catholic. At this stage of the game, I don't want to upset her, so I just go along with it. I never told her about Marge, not that I have anything to hide. I just like to keep it to myself, something that's a part of both of us. I don't want to spill it around. She was too precious to be talking about just anywhere.

I'll die loving her. You love someone, and through your own stupidity it's taken away from you. You only meet someone like that once in a lifetime, and I was so stupid I couldn't see it. Nothing to do about it now. It's done.

I'm getting weaker and weaker. Maybe I'll just sleep. And maybe that's it. All my affairs are in order. I took care of that before I came into hospital. It wasn't much to get in order. I don't have much.

I'm a bit nervous about the thought of dying. I don't know why. Yes, I'm a bit nervous about it. Who wouldn't be? I have no idea at all what will happen. I never thought about it till now. No idea at all. Everyone is on an equal footing there, I guess. I'd have to be ready when it comes. Nothing to be done now. Don't have the strength to do much anyway. Can't do much else but sleep. Maybe I'll just slip into it without having to prepare or be nervous. The old pendulum will come back to normal again, it'll straighten itself out. Like always. Why would death be any different from life?

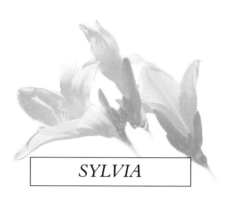

SYLVIA

I got Sylvia's name from the ALS *society as someone who was very willing to talk. On the phone, we made an appointment, and she gave me directions to her house. She lived in the suburbs on a tree-lined crescent filled with modern houses. Her door was opened by a Philippine woman, who led me into the living room to where Sylvia was seated calmly in a chair with a blanket over her legs. Her hands lay still on the arms of the chair. Her brown hair fell in soft curls to her shoulders. At thirty-six, she was attractive and elegant. Later I realized that the blanket over her legs was meant to hide any deformity that might have been caused by her inability to use her leg muscles. And she probably no longer had any control over her hands, which she never moved throughout our numerous interviews.*

During our talks she was full of poise, and her manner was admirably contained. Even when she talked about the difficult areas of her life, I could tell that they were simply memories that she had already worked through and was now merely relating.

Whenever I visited, the Philippine woman opened the door and showed me in. Sylvia sat in place, in her chair, beside a small table. She was always in a good mood, welcoming this opportunity to talk. She was a very even-tempered person who exuded a certain calm, who had found answers to life that satisfied her, and who was no

longer searching, asking questions. Even so, she was more than open
to other possibilities and carefully considered any connections that I
made from one interview to the next.

I always said, "I want to die in a car accident, something quick. I
don't want to suffer." But this disease is not physically painful. I look
sick, I don't feel sick. My body is changing, diminishing in capacity,
but what's a body? You only need it for certain things. Right now it
houses my mind which flourishes while the structure degenerates.
Soon it will totally collapse.

I wrote in my will that I don't want to be kept alive by a respirator. It would be painful for my kids to see me connected to machines.
I want death to be a natural end. I don't want to artificially extend
my life, nor do I want to end it before its time. Though I believe if
people are tired of being sick, they have the freedom to end their life.
I don't think God expects to have full control. We are given control,
and it's for us to take it.

Every life is complete, no matter when or how a person dies. I
believe we come in here to learn and to teach others. When babies
die a crib death or when children die young, I think they have just
come in to teach their parents something. When I will die, I will have
learned what I needed to learn, and my illness and death will have
taught others, like my daughters. I don't exactly know what my illness has to teach them, but I'm sure there is something.

To date, this disease has taught me to value myself and has shown
me that I'm a fighter. It's a paradox. I gain inner strength as my physical capacities diminish. I don't think about the illness twenty-four
hours a day, I can transcend it. I fight to live with a smile and with
my spirits intact. I don't want my daughters to see me weak. I fight
to give them my best, in spite of my condition. They know I'm sick,
of course, but I don't want them to say, Oh, my mother is sick. I want
them to say, My mother is sick but she is strong.

At school, the teacher asked Stephanie's class, "What would you
do if you found out you had cancer and you'll soon die?"

Stephanie was the first to answer. She said, "I'll be like my mother, I'll continue to fight with a smile."

If they remember me with a smile, I will have done my job. Sometimes I get angry, like all mothers, but I don't want to get depressed. I don't want to let myself go. I'm not in my bedroom all the time. My helper bathes and dresses me every morning and takes me out to the living room, which is totally open and gives me a view of the kitchen, the front entrance, and the whole length of the house. This allows me to participate in life.

Before, I thought I participated in life, but the quality of that participation was totally different. Before, I only tried to please others. And I felt that nothing I did was ever enough. When I was in school and showed my mother my report card, it was never good enough. The way I looked wasn't good enough. She used to say, "Eat, eat, you're too thin."

When I was thirteen, I didn't have any breasts, and she bought me a padded bra to wear. She said I had to be sexy. When I was fourteen or fifteen we often went shopping together, and she used to say, very pleased and proud, "All the men look at you." I didn't understand why, I didn't think I was pretty.

I usually did what my mother told me to do, partly because when you're young you think your mother is right, and she was very authoritarian. It was impossible to question or contradict her. Plus, I could only please her by doing what she wanted.

Later I did things to please Mark. And, again, it was never enough. From the time we began to go out, he always watched what I ate. He told me how to dress, how to do my hair when we went out. He was always trying to control me. Before we got married, he said, "If you become as fat as your mother, I'll divorce you."

After we got married, he never complimented me on anything. I kept trying harder and harder to please him, and I never could. He never said, You're a good cook. Or, You have good taste.

CB

Mark and I met when I was sixteen and he was eighteen. At the time, he was already studying mathematics at McGill University. After we had known each other for a few months, he said, "I have a heavy course load. I'm going to have to study really hard if I want good grades and a lucrative future. I like you, but I can only see you Friday night and Saturday night. If you can accept that, we'll go out, and I won't see anyone else."

I said, "Fine." I loved him. He was serious, solid, mature.

My mother thought Mark was the perfect man. She said, "Stay with him. One day he's going to make good money."

Whenever I told her about an argument we had, she said, "Be careful, no other man will take you seriously now. You're lucky he still wants you." She was convinced no other men would want me because we had made love and I wasn't a virgin. And this was the 1980s.

Mark finished university at twenty-one. After he graduated, we got married. I was nineteen. He got a good job with a major corporation, then went back to university at night for his MBA. During the day, I was a receptionist in a law firm. I had friends at work but didn't see them in the evening. At night, I cooked supper for the two of us and watched TV. He was always studying, which didn't bother me. He said he was working for our future, to make good money, to build a secure life.

However, I often dreamed of Mark having affairs with other women. Very often. It really upset me. I couldn't understand it. I woke up in the morning feeling depressed. I said to him, "You're always cheating on me in my dreams."

He laughed. "Was she cute?"

On weekends, when we went dancing or to a restaurant, he made me walk a few steps ahead of him so he could see how many people were looking at me. I didn't even notice it, my friends pointed it out to me. When men made comments about me at a party, Mark never said, That's my wife, watch what you say. He just listened. He liked to hear what other men said about me. He was proud when they made comments about my looks.

Because I knew my looks were important to Mark, I always paid attention to my appearance. Every day, first thing in the morning, I put on mascara, eyeliner, blush, lipstick. If I was wearing red, I put on red nail polish, if I was wearing pink I put on pink nail polish, if I was wearing something orange, I had orange nail polish. I changed my nail polish every day to go with my outfit. I was always well dressed, even when going to the corner store. I never wore jeans.

Three years after we were married, I got pregnant. He was furious. We had been careful, and my getting pregnant was an accident. He wanted me to get an abortion.

I said, "Why? We have everything. We have a good life, you have a high salary, a stable job." He was a treasurer at a corporation and doing very well. I didn't see any reason to have an abortion. Plus we had talked about having children. When we got married, I told him I wanted a family, and he had agreed. I didn't want a career, I didn't want to study. I didn't have big expectations for myself. I wanted to stay home and have a family. I loved kids when I was young. I babysat every day till the summer before I got married. But Mark said he didn't want children at this point. When I spoke to my mother about his reaction to my pregnancy, she took his side. She blamed me for getting pregnant.

I told him I wanted to keep the baby. He said he didn't want our life to change because of the child. He didn't want me to gain weight. But, of course, as the child grew inside me I got bigger and bigger, and he refused to take me out because of my size.

I said to myself, "I'll show both my mother and Mark that I'm strong, I can have what I want. I want a daughter, and I will have a daughter."

I didn't want to give birth to a boy, to another Mark. Before, I never thought about what I wanted. I only thought of pleasing my mother and then pleasing Mark. When I got pregnant, I started to think about myself. I loved being pregnant. It made me feel important. I was creating a human life. I took excellent care of myself. No smoking. No alcohol. No junk food. I wanted to create the best environment for this growing baby inside me. I was very protective toward it, which made me become more assertive. For the first time in my life, if I didn't want to do something, I didn't do it. Mark wasn't pleased about the change. He was losing control over me.

The day before Stephanie was born, he said, "I'm not ready to be a father."

I gave birth on a Wednesday, and the next Friday he wanted to go out dancing and told me not to wear my pregnancy clothes. I said, "Mark, I'm still big, I can't wear regular clothes yet." It was terrible. I wouldn't wish it on anyone.

After Stephanie was born, I became more vocal. And we were always fighting. It's your turn. No, it's your turn. For five years we woke up every night. Either she wanted her bottle or a kiss, a hug, scratch my back, had a bad dream, needed to be covered up. Every night there was something. We took her to his mother's on weekends so we could sleep.

Stephanie was the kind of baby who had a tantrum whenever she couldn't get what she wanted. If you said no to her, she started yelling and screaming. Every time she had a fit of anger, Mark blamed me for it. He kept telling me to be more patient with her. Finally I lost my temper. I said to him, "Who do you think you are, telling me what to wear, what to eat, where to go, how to raise my child?" And I changed my married name back to my maiden name. He didn't like that.

After a year, I said, "I want to spend more time with my daughter. We have enough money, I'm going to work three days a week."

Once a week, I took aerobics classes and then went to have dinner with friends. He had his night off to play hockey, and I had my night off. It was wonderful. For the first time in my life, I felt free. But we were always arguing over Stephanie. If I said no to her, he said yes. If I said yes, he said no. If I said white, he said black. All the time. Even now.

Because he realized he was losing control over me, he used Stephanie to put me down, to contradict me. He gave her whatever she wanted, even if against my wishes. He wanted to show me that what I thought and wanted didn't count. If I suggested we go see *Snow White* and Stephanie wanted to see *Pinocchio*, he said, "If she wants to see *Pinocchio*, we'll see *Pinocchio*."

If I said I didn't feel like cooking, she said, "We'll call Daddy and he'll pick up some food on his way home." If I would ask him, he'd say no. If she asked him, he did it. He never says no to her, never, never. He never tells her what to do, what to eat, or what to wear. She knows exactly what she wants, and he lets her have it. She's not at all like I was, trying to please, trying to adapt, be nice.

I used to smoke, and one day Mark said, "If you stop smoking, I'll buy you a fur coat." He thought people who smoked were crass, low class.

I stopped smoking for a few years, then started again behind his back. Five years ago, we went out to dinner with three other couples. The men were Mark's colleagues. After a few drinks, the women said, "Sylvia, come with us. We're going to the bathroom to fix our makeup."

In the bathroom, all the women lit up a cigarette. They, too, had to hide from their husbands, and some of them were forty and fifty. I was the youngest of the four. I felt like a teenager smoking in the bathroom. I thought, We're crazy. We're doing everything the men want because they have the money and presume they also have the control.

After that I began to smoke in front of Mark. That created a lot of fights. He said I smelled and tasted like an ashtray. We made love, and he refused to kiss me. I refused to stop smoking. I stood up for myself.

He tried to exercise his control in other areas as well. Chips, for instance. He didn't want me to eat chips because he didn't want me to gain weight. And I love chips. I had to hide the bags and eat them on the sly, when he wasn't home. He got angry when he saw me snacking at night. Neither did he tolerate eating between meals. Once in Barbados we took a long walk and came to a place that sold delicious-looking french fries. I was tired and hungry. I had left my wallet back home because I hadn't expected to go on such a long walk. I asked Mark to buy me some fries. He said, "Why? It's not dinner time." He wouldn't buy me any.

Pizza was another issue. He didn't want me to order pizza. He didn't want a pizza delivery truck seen in front of the house. He said,

"My mother never ordered ready-made food. Only poor people have food delivered to the house."

I could have picked up the pizza, that would have been all right. Instead of having an argument all the time, I burned the boxes. Sometimes he worked late and I ordered a pizza. I ate it, put the pizza box in the toilet bowl, and lit it. No proof. Even when Stephanie suggested we order pizza, he said, "No, I'll go and pick it up."

For the first five years after Stephanie's birth, we didn't want another child because she was taking up so much time and energy. When she started school, she was busy and required much less attention. At that point I said to him, "I want a second child, but this time you make the decision when. I don't want to go through what we went through the first time. But there is a limit. I want a second child before I'm thirty."

For a while things were fine between us. When we were on vacation in Florida, he said, "I think it's the right time to have another baby, and you can stop working to take care of the kids. But don't expect me to get up during the night for the feeding. You'll have to take care of both yourself."

That's exactly what I wanted. So when I was twenty-nine, we tried for a baby. It worked the first try. I was thrilled. He said, "I hope you don't get as big as the last time." Two months later, I miscarried, I'm sure because of what he had said. But I got pregnant again soon after.

When I got the pregnancy results, I called him at work and said, "Meet me at Thursday's after work. I have some news."

Sometimes he liked to meet for a drink after work. I always arrived before him, and when he came in he had to look all around the room to find me. I liked that. I think he also liked it. That night, when I told him I was pregnant again, was the last time we met for a drink.

The first pregnancy was easy. The second one was very difficult. After two months, I began to bleed. I was due to give birth in October, and a month later I would have turned thirty. I thought this was my last chance. I didn't want to lose the baby. After twenty weeks of pregnancy, I was bleeding so much I had to go to the hospital for four days. The doctor told me to rest. I was on my back for most of the pregnancy and had to go into hospital five more times. I was bleeding the full term. At one point, in the hospital, I told the nurses I probably had a boy because only men can give you so much trouble. And I wanted to have a second daughter.

One night I was taking two plates of spaghetti from the kitchen counter to the table for Stephanie, and the strength went out of my left arm. The plate of spaghetti just fell out of my hand and onto the floor. I thought it strange, but I paid no attention. I thought I was tired because I was having such a hard pregnancy, and I was afraid of losing the baby.

I gave birth to Virginia after thirty weeks. It was an emergency C-section, and she weighed three pounds. After the birth, I found some movements hard to do with my left arm. When I looked at myself in the mirror, my left shoulder looked as if it was getting thinner. And I was always tired. If I did the laundry, I didn't have the energy to do anything else that day. I didn't understand it. I couldn't blame Virginia because after delivery she had stayed in hospital for six weeks. That should have given me enough time to recover. And when she came home, she was a very good baby. She was quiet, slept through the night.

I thought something must be wrong with me. I went to see an orthopedist because one of my friends suggested I might have problems with my joints. The orthopedist sent me to a neurologist, who gave me an EMG and said, "Just take some physio and you'll get better." I began taking physio. When the insurance stopped paying for it, I had to quit. Mark refused to pay. I was really upset. We certainly had the money.

I had a hard summer because I was afraid something was wrong with me and didn't know what. Mark paid no attention to me. He came home from work after the kids were in bed. I wanted him to come home earlier and spend some evenings with me. I was feeling very nervous and needed some emotional support.

He said, "I don't have time for hand-holding. I have to work. Call a friend."

"I don't need a friend. I need you."

He just couldn't understand. When I told him I was worried something was wrong with me, he said, "Don't worry, you're probably just tired. But why are you tired? You're hardly doing anything. The house is a mess."

At one point, I thought he was the cause of whatever was wrong. I believe every illness has a reason. Usually an unconscious one. Perhaps I thought if I got sick he would give me more of his time. But he was never there before and wasn't going to be there any more just because I was sick.

He wasn't very attentive to Virginia, either. Once he took Stephanie somewhere and left Virginia crying and yelling in the middle of the street, "Daddy, you forgot to take me."

My neighbour brought her inside. He often left without Virginia, even if he just went to pick up milk. He said he didn't want to take both girls. I said, "If you don't want to take them both, don't take either."

It was like talking to a wall. He would be hiding from her, pretending to be in his office when he went to the garage to start the car. And she's not stupid.

One night, four years ago, I was watching a program on wife abuse, and it really touched a nerve. At first I couldn't understand why I had such a profound reaction. As I thought about it, I realized I, too, was being abused psychologically. I was angry at myself for having allowed it to happen, for not having been quick enough to notice it before. I had time alone to think about what I was watching before Mark came in toward the end of the program. His immediate reaction was, "Why are you watching such rubbish?"

I told him I thought he was abusing me.

He laughed. He said I was easily influenced. But the program was like a switch that had gone on. It was a revelation.

In the meantime, my symptoms were not going away. That fall, I went back to see the same neurologist. He gave me another EMG and said, "Something has changed. We'll have to do more tests."

I asked, "Why?"

He said, "I think you have a brain tumour."

"I can't have a brain tumour, I don't have any symptoms. I don't have trouble with my balance or sight. I have no headaches."

"That doesn't matter."

After two weeks of tests in the hospital, he said, "Your motor neurons are dying and can no longer communicate with your muscles. You have a brain tumour." Just like that, no compassion, no support, no warmth. After I left the hospital, I said, "I don't want to see him again."

I went to another neurologist, who gave me another EMG and said whatever I had will go just as it had come. I didn't think he was right. I went to a third neurologist, who said I had muscular dystrophy.

Then Mark talked about me to his doctor who set up an appointment with a neurologist known to specialize in my symptoms. I went to see him, and he was very kind. He listened to me, answered my questions. And he wanted to give me another EMG. This was to be my fourth, and the procedure is very painful. They put at least twenty-five needles in different muscles and move the needles around while checking the machine. This time, when the doctor started to put in the needles, I began to shake and cry uncontrollably. Partly because the disease I have affects the muscles and the nervous system. When I'm nervous, I become breathless and all emotions are exaggerated, which is odd because it's always been hard for me to express my emotions. I think for most of my life I didn't even allow myself to feel my own emotions. I was too eager to please other people. Now my own emotions force themselves upon me, sometimes rather vehemently.

When I finally managed to calm down, I said, "I can't take this anymore."

The doctor patted my shoulder, "We have something to calm you."

I asked, "Can you give me something so I won't feel any pain at all?"

"Of course."

During the test, I felt nothing. I had had three earlier tests at three different hospitals, and no one said I could have it pain-free. During one test I was crying and swearing, and I never swear. When the test was over, I apologized to the doctor, who said, "I'm used to it."

I also had to have an operation. My leg was opened up to remove a part of a muscle for tests. I asked Mark to be with me after the operation. He said, "Why?"

I then called a girlfriend. He came to visit for five minutes. That's it.

When all the tests were done, the doctor told me I had ALS, amyotrophic lateral sclerosis. Mark's uncle had died of the same disease eight years earlier. I remember neither he nor his mother could cry at his funeral. His mother never wanted to talk about him or his disease after his death.

When I heard what I had, my first fear was death and the thought that my daughters might have inherited this same disease. The doctor clearly explained to me what to expect, the degeneration of the muscles till finally I wouldn't be able to do anything. The throat and heart muscles will also cease and will probably be the cause of death. Lifespan, after diagnosis, differs with the individual. He said doing physiotherapy can slow down the degeneration.

Two weeks later, I began to do physio and continued to do it twice a week for one year and once a week for two more years. There were a lot of physiotherapists at the hospital, and I chose Lisa. We immediately started talking about spiritual things like a higher power, reincarnation, visualization. The only other person I had such conversations with was my chiropractor, who used to say we all find what we need. And I needed Lisa at that time. The relationship I had with her, both as a therapist and as a friend, gave me hope and strength. She never judged me. Sometimes I went to the hospital feeling very low. She immediately sensed it. A few times we didn't do any exercises at all because I was crying too much, and she allowed me to simply cry. I once had a pain in my shoulder and she gave me a Reiki treatment. The pain immediately disappeared.

Also, she gave me keys to open my mind. She made me a forty-five minute relaxation and visualization tape. I listened to it every night before going to sleep. It really helped me. Mark hated it. I wouldn't allow him to talk or move in bed while I was listening to it.

ob

At first, I had problems lifting my left arm, then the right arm, but I could still drive and walk. Soon I had problems climbing the first step along the walkway leading to the house. I asked Mark to have a small ramp installed. He paid no attention. One night, when we came home from his parents', I lost my balance going up the step and fell on the pavement. My head began to bleed badly, and Mark had to take me to hospital for stitches. I was crying all the way there. I thought, I'm thirty-two years old and I'm going to lose the use of my legs. In the waiting room of the hospital, he said to me, "Stop crying, everyone is staring at you."

When we went into the doctor's office, he said, "I hope this won't take long. I haven't had dinner yet, and I'm starving."

I thought, He doesn't care about me at all. I split my head, I'm getting stitches, and I'm in pain.

At around this time, my neighbour, who had babysat Stephanie for three years and who was also a friend, died in a car accident while her husband escaped with only a broken arm. When I heard about it, I cried and thought, Why didn't I die? I'm the one who's sick. She was healthy. Then I thought, Why didn't her husband die? She was always running around, always the one to take her three sons skiing or bike riding or to play tennis. Plus she babysat all the kids on the street. Her husband spent his spare time reading in the back yard.

A few weeks before she died, she told me she was tired of doing everything and resented her husband for never lifting a finger to help.

Mark and I went to the funeral home. It was ugly and depressing. It was all sombre inside, plus I hated the wallpaper. I told him I didn't want to end up there when I died. And I thought I should probably visit some funeral homes to choose which one I wanted.

That was the last time I went to a funeral home or to a funeral. Emotionally, it was just too difficult for me. My aunt and uncle died last summer, and I didn't go. Mark's grandfather died and I didn't go. The father of one of my best friends died, and I didn't go. I don't want to go because I'll start sobbing uncontrollably, and it wouldn't be over the person who has just died but for myself. I'm not afraid to die, but at a funeral I see what it'll be like when I'm dead, not with me in the coffin, but with the people around me. Everyone crying, sad.

Before I got sick, I had a dream that I was dead in a coffin. People were standing around me and crying. I remember saying to them, "Don't cry, I feel great." I think when I'll be dead that's exactly what I'll say to them. "Maybe you'll cry because you'll miss me, but don't worry about where I am or what I'm doing. I'm fine."

Now, I sometimes sit in the living room, look out at this neighbour's house, and think perhaps she's sitting on the roof, protecting her sons and husband.

After I fell on the pavement and had to have stitches in my head, I began to have problems walking. I had to get a walker. But can you imagine walking to the bathroom with a walker after you just made love? Totally nude. I couldn't do it. Making love and the walker didn't go together. After we made love, I asked Mark to help me to the bathroom. He always made such a fuss. He didn't want to help me. He refused. Can you imagine? And we had just made love a minute ago. I didn't say a word, I just cried. I was very, very upset. Sometimes he said, "We'll make love, but I don't want you to go to the bathroom after."

I said, "You go to the bathroom afterwards. I have the same needs." I thought, Why can't he at least take care of one part of me? There are two women in me. I'm a woman and I'm handicapped. If you don't want to help me because I'm handicapped, I understand. But he didn't want to take care of me as a woman, either.

I couldn't take it anymore and finally said, "If you don't want to help me to the bathroom, we won't make love." I thought he might say, I'll help you, don't worry.

Instead he said, "Then we won't make love." And we stopped making love. He no longer kissed me, never hugged me. And stopped paying any attention to me.

I think when I could no longer walk by myself I was finished for

Mark. I was no good. He has never helped me. He has never really been there for much of anything, I realize. When I was well, he never came with us to the movies, the circus, shopping. He thought all that was boring. He never helped us decorate the Christmas tree. He said it was a waste of a tree. I loved to decorate the tree with the girls. I even put lights in the windows. For Easter, I put out bunnies and baskets of Easter eggs. I made special dinners. This year, on Valentine's Day, I said to the girls, let's dress up in red for the day. Mark just couldn't appreciate it.

At one point I began to see a psychologist. I wanted to discuss my feelings about the illness. It turned out that the disease was not my main problem. It was Mark. After a time, the psychologist suggested the two of us see someone who worked with couples.

Mark found out the company would pay for twelve weeks of therapy and agreed to come with me. He didn't want to pay for it himself. We went to see a psychologist for the first time together two and a half years ago. She gave us exercises to do. She also had us ask each other questions. I asked Mark, "Why are you so cold? Unfeeling?"

He didn't answer. When the therapist asked him how he felt, all he could say was that he was very sad.

Also, she had us communicate with each other through her. I said, "I would have thought you would be more loving as I got sick, but you weren't. I didn't want to change you. I just wanted you to show some affection." He said, "You expect too much of me. I can't fulfill your expectations. I've already done more than I should have."

When you can't do something by yourself and someone has to help you, but he's not paying attention and does it wrong, it can be very frustrating. When I started to have difficulty walking or standing up, I had to ask Mark to help. I gave him my hand and said, "Wait a minute, I'll tell you when. I'm not ready to stand up yet. I need to get my balance first."

But he wasn't listening. He just pulled me up, and most of the time I fell. And I was angry, I was yelling at him. With this disease you're totally dependent on other people to help you, and if the person closest to you doesn't make the effort to pay attention and is always complaining when you ask for something, it can be infuriating. When we were eating, I sometimes asked him to cut my food. He said, "Cut it yourself."

"But I can't."

"At least try."

Now Virginia cuts my food most of the time. She says, "We'll play, Mummy, you're the baby and I'm the mother." And she feeds me.

I let my daughters help with simple things. I don't want them to help me walk. They're young and not very strong. If I were to fall while they're helping me, they would blame themselves. And it wouldn't be their fault, it would be mine. But try to explain that to a child.

One day I fell on the floor, and Stephanie called Mark at work. She said, "Come right away! Mummy is on the floor, she can't get up by herself."

He came home around four-thirty and said, "Next time don't disturb me at the office for such nonsense. Find someone else."

My mother came two days a week to do all the shopping and cooking. Mark's mother and father were here every Sunday for a year so he wouldn't have to do anything in the house. Two years ago, I thought, I need someone to help me. Though I could still go to the bathroom by myself, I could no longer do much else. The first time I mentioned needing someone to help, Mark objected. He said it was too expensive. As I continued to ask him to scratch my back and do little things here and there, he soon realized there was no choice but to get someone. At around that time, Louise, a friend of mine, was laid off work and offered to help. She came five days a week and stayed till six in the evening. I wanted Mark to be home as soon as possible after Louise left for the day because I was scared to be home alone for too long. Once Virginia was crying in the middle of the street, and I couldn't go out to see what was wrong. I was powerless to do anything. It was a terrible feeling. But he was annoyed at having to come home so early. He was always complaining that he couldn't finish his work at the office.

In October, Mark announced that he was very tired and his performance at work was suffering. He went to live in a hotel for four months. He came home on weekends, but it wasn't very pleasant because I was so upset by the whole arrangement.

Louise, since she was a friend, became too involved in my private life. When Mark left, I was very depressed, and it was hard to be with me. After helping me for a year, she decided she wanted to find another type of job. When she left, I insisted that Mark come back. Two or three weeks later, a neighbour's live-in help was let go, and she came to ask me if I needed someone. It was perfect timing. We set up the spare room for her, and she came to live with us. That was a very convenient arrangement for Mark. He could come home as late as he wanted because he knew she was with me. And he stayed away more and more.

A year later, in therapy, Mark and I started to talk about a separation. In September, he began looking for an apartment, then stopped. It was already November and soon it would be Christmas. A separation two weeks before Christmas would be hard on the kids, so I didn't push him to continue looking for an apartment. Then, out of the blue, he said, "I don't want to leave."

"Why do you want to stay? You don't touch me. You don't talk to me. You ignore me. I don't look as attractive as before, so why stay with me?"

He said, "I'm not leaving."

"Why?"

"I don't want to leave."

By now I needed to use a wheelchair when going outside and used a walker indoors. But when you get inside the house, there are about ten stair-steps leading from the foyer to the main floor. It became harder and harder for me to walk up the stairs with a walker. I asked Mark to install a chair lift along the stairs from the entrance to the first floor. He said, "No, it's too expensive." Two weeks later, Stephanie asked for braces, and he said, "Fine."

Because I couldn't climb the stairs I didn't go out. I realized that if I wanted to continue living, I needed that chair. I had a little money of my own and decided to pay for it myself. I called and arranged to have a chair lift installed. When he saw it he said I had wasted my money.

The next day, my mother came over to help me. The woman who lived with us was out shopping. And I fell while she was gone. My mother tried to lift me, and I fell again. She finally called the police. When Mark came home from work my mother was crying. She said to him, "Sylvia fell on the floor and I had to call the police. I was so nervous."

Mark just shrugged. No sympathy. No compassion. That was a Wednesday. The following Monday, I called the lawyer and said, "I want him out of here."

At the next therapy session, which took place in the house, I said to him, "You'll have to look for an apartment."

He said, "I'm staying here."

I said, "You'll have to leave. On January 10 you'll receive a lawyer's letter asking you to leave. I don't want you here anymore."

He said nothing. He didn't think I was serious. I thought, "Let him stay for Christmas, and he can leave in the New Year."

There is a New Year's Day tradition in my family that's very important to me. The oldest child asks the father to bless the family. And I'm the oldest. As long as my father is alive and I'm alive, I'll ask him to bless us. My father, being the eldest of his family, used to ask his father to bless everyone. But one year he couldn't visit his father to ask for the blessing, and my grandfather died on January 10. This left a strong impression on him. I was only three at the time, and he has repeated the story to me several times since. This year, on New Year's Day, when we were all at my parents' house, I waited till Mark went to the bathroom before I asked for my father's blessing, and I asked him to exclude Mark. By then my family knew we were going to separate.

Before Mark left, I wanted to know what he looked for in a woman. He said, "Someone who doesn't smoke, is attractive, and independent."

Everything I'm not. That hurt. I loved him for so many years. I invested my hopes and dreams in this man. My life. I would have done anything for him. And when I needed him the most, he wasn't there. In a sense, his coldness and lack of attention pushed me to discover my own strength. Now I no longer need him.

After the separation, we had one more session with the psychologist. I asked Mark if he felt anything. Here I was, a handicapped woman with two children, and I happen to be his wife and the children are his daughters. And he left them. Did he feel sad, mad, anything?

He said, "No, nothing, I can't allow my feelings to interfere with my performance at work."

He puts all his energy into work because he thinks everything has a price. I said, "I hope you lose your job. It would be the best thing for you."

He was shocked. "If I lose my job, you won't have any money."

"I don't need money." I think it would be the lesson of his life, especially today when it's so hard to find a job.

My daughters and I are staying in the house he worked so hard to buy. We bought it thirteen years ago and had it painted before moving in. But did nothing more to it. I didn't want to spend money on the house because I was never here. What's the point of buying and fixing things when you're not around to enjoy them? When I became sick and was forced to stay home, I had all the rooms re-painted. I had the kitchen renovated. I arranged everything the way I wanted. I really made the house my own. When Mark left, I didn't allow him to take anything. I said, "That's the price of your freedom. For you, everything has a price. Freedom also has a price."

He left with only a suitcase full of clothes.

Would I have stayed with him if I wouldn't have become ill? Would I have put up with him for the rest of my life? I don't know. Before I became sick Mark didn't pay any attention to my feelings. The illness certainly didn't make him any more caring or affectionate. But I became more aware of my own need for affection and warmth, something I had denied myself most of my life. And I feel this awareness has made me a better person. It has allowed me to see with greater clarity. I said earlier that my physiotherapist gave me keys to open my mind. The illness has done exactly the same thing.

I cried more when Mark left than when I found out I had ALS. I cried for three weeks after he was gone. Not three months or three years, three weeks. I was depressed because Mark stepping out of my life meant the end of something familiar. It meant the end of a family. It was odd. A part of me wanted him out of my life while another part of me mourned the end of a dream that could never have been. Not with him.

I was never depressed because of the illness. After I received the diagnosis, I made a conscious decision not to be depressed. If I'm depressed, no one will want to see me or be with me. I would find myself very alone. And I have a lot of good friends who I like and need. If one is busy, I know I can call another one. I need them, but they also need me. They know they can come here any time to talk about their problems. I'm always here, and they won't disturb me. I can't help physically, but I can help emotionally.

Now my sister-in-law is very depressed. Three months ago, Mark's brother left her with a sixteen-month-old baby. She's still crying. I told her not to make herself sick, he's not worth it. Remember all the bad things he did, and you'll be grateful he left.

The odd time when I still cry about Mark I just say to myself, Don't waste your tears, you lost nothing of value. I cry when I remember the good times, and of course there were good times. Now I talk to him on the phone almost every day. He calls either about the girls or money arrangements, and he never asks how I am. When he comes to pick up the kids, he stays outside. I can't see him. Seeing him makes me very angry. Of course, he doesn't care whether he sees me or not, and even over the phone he treats me as he has always done. When Stephanie throws a tantrum and I have to call to ask him to calm her, his immediate response is, "What did you do to her?" It's my fault. He still always takes Stephanie's side. Now she's twelve, and she thinks whenever she asks for something she'll get it. Since

Mark left in January, I'm starting to say no to her and she gets angry. One night, soon after he left, I didn't let her watch TV, and she said, "I'll kill you. You're just a crippled woman." She was terrible.

Now when I say no to her, she's mad, but she no longer says such rude things.

Unlike Mark, who refused to change, the disease is always changing, progressing, developing. Mark is gone, the disease is here to stay. My body is visibly deteriorating while my mind is becoming clearer and clearer. But sometimes I mourn the things I can no longer do. Virginia, who is now five, will sometimes say, "Do you remember when we once went bicycling?"

She was no more than two or three at the time, and she still remembers. Or she'll ask, "Do you remember when you used to drive?" I haven't driven for two years. Or if she sees me on videos she'll say, "Hey, you weren't handicapped then! One day you won't be handicapped anymore, Mom, and we'll go bicycling."

That made me cry because I know I'm not a normal mother. I can't go with her to school activities. I can't play with her. Still, I do the best I can.

Now I have everything I need to go out. A wheelchair, a lift that takes me down the stairs, a ramp leading from the front door to the street. Last week it was sunny, and I said to Virginia, "I'll go in the wheelchair, you take your bicycle, and we'll drive around."

She was so happy. It was simple fun. I do what I can. She knows that and accepts it. When someone asks her about me, she says, "My mother is in a wheelchair because she's handicapped." She's not ashamed of it. Stephanie was ashamed of me. When I began to go out in a wheelchair, she didn't want to walk beside me. Now she's more comfortable with it. But she still gets angry from time to time and says, "I hate to see you in a wheelchair." Having said that, she feels better.

For Stephanie this reality, with me sick, is hard. She doesn't accept my illness because she remembers what it was like before, when I was always on the run and took her with me everywhere. I went to see friends, family, went shopping, out to eat. Monday I went to the market. Tuesday I had dinner at my mother's. Wednesday I played badminton, then had dinner with friends. I had something to do every day. I was running all the time. Dress Stephanie. Undress her. All the time. Stephanie remembers the running around. She said, "Do you remember, Mom, we were never home?"

She was right. After Virginia everything changed.

One night, Stephanie said, "Virginia will never know what it's like to have a real mother." Virginia didn't know me when I was healthy. I've been sick ever since she was born. She comes back from friends' houses and says, "My friends' mothers work so hard. They're always rushing around and tired." She pities them. She's never seen me work.

After Mark left, Stephanie once said to me, "You do nothing all day. You're always sitting in this chair watching TV."

I said, "Look at the good side. I'm always here for you."

She said, "All the other mothers work. Why don't you? You should find a job."

I said, "I have a job already, I'm raising you kids."

"That's not a job. You don't earn any money."

I said, "You should be glad your mother is here when you leave for school and when you come home."

The other day she said, "I hate Daddy for what he did."

Now she talks about not wanting to see him, and I think it's my fault because sometimes I talk negatively about Mark in front of her, and I shouldn't. I have to be careful. If I'm mad at Mark, she'll also be mad at him. She said, "I feel like a slice of ham between two pieces of bread." I was surprised. She said, "When I'm with you, you're mad at Daddy and then I'm mad at Daddy, and when I'm with Daddy, he doesn't want to hear about you, so we can't mention you. Virginia and I don't know what to do."

I told her I wasn't angry at her father anymore and she shouldn't be either.

Stephanie started her period shortly after her twelfth birthday, the weekend after Mark left. She cried when she got it. She said it smelled bad and she didn't want it. I said, "You have no choice. That's one of the things in life you can't control." I keep telling her there are things she can't control, like the weather. She thinks she can have everything she wants. Maybe she has to learn the hard way.

She's smart like Mark and is one year ahead in school because she skipped a grade. Since she's with older kids, she feels superior. She's in a class with fourteen- and fifteen-year-olds, and one girl is pregnant. Now she wants to have a boyfriend, and I won't let her have one at twelve. She gets angry.

Right now Stephanie doesn't like life very much. She thinks everything is stupid. School isn't worth anything. Life isn't worth anything. Only friendship has value. And she's talking about suicide. I've read that when kids really want to kill themselves, they have a plan, and Stephanie has no plan. I think she just wants attention. She said, "I'm going to kill myself. I'm going to throw myself out the window."

I said, "You won't kill yourself that way. You'll just break a leg."

She's trying to see if I'm going to cry or protest. Once we watched a TV program on teenage suicide, and she asked me, "Would you be sad if I died?"

I said, "Of course, but if you think you'll be happier dead, it's your choice. If you stood before me with a gun pointed at your head, I would try to stop you, but you know I couldn't even do that because I can't use my hands." I am trying to give her tools to help her deal with her problems. There is nothing more I can do.

Sometimes my mother says things like, "I'm afraid Stephanie will end up sleeping on the street. She'll do drugs. She'll become a prostitute." My mother likes melodrama. She watches too much TV. I said, "What do you want me to do?" She seemed to insinuate that it would be my fault if these things should happen. Everything is my fault. Even after I had asked Mark to leave, she said it was my fault that he had left.

My mother is a master at blaming others for all sorts of things, both real and imaginary, and at complaining about everything. Before I was sick, I let her talk on. Now, when it becomes too much, I tell her to stop. She watches all the talk shows. She likes to read about actors, actresses, singers. The life of the stars is part of her conversation, like they are her intimate friends. Talk to her about something that has nothing to do with the stars and she's not interested. When I called her up to tell her I was pregnant, she said, "By the way, Liza Minnelli lost her baby yesterday."

Now, when I'm tired, I say, "Don't talk to me about trivialities. I don't care. I don't want to know." Before, I couldn't do that. But when she comes here I still get breathless. She's always moving, finding things to do that don't need doing. She can't sit still. She's hyperactive. I told my father she should be on something to calm her.

Two weeks before Easter, I asked my mother not to buy me anything. No flowers, no chocolates, nothing. I just want them to come over for dinner. Of course, she brought me flowers and a gift. Inside the box was a little plaster angel. She said I needed it as my guardian angel. I said, "I already have a guardian angel."

"Where is it?"

"You can't see it." I gave the gift back to her. I know she felt bad. But I don't want her to spend money on foolish things, especially since I know they aren't well off. I would prefer a hug.

Since I'm sick, my mother has never hugged me. My father, yes, not my mother. And I wish she would give me emotional support instead of always criticism.

My mother doesn't know how to be supportive and neither does my twenty-year-old sister. The last time I saw her was Christmas. She has called me once since Mark left. On the phone, I told her he had moved into an expensive apartment. She said, "Did you expect him to live in a basement while you keep that big house?"

I said, "You're my sister, you're supposed to take my side."

When I asked her to come over, she said, "I don't have time." I called her a week later to invite her again. She said, "Seeing you unable to move makes me want to cry."

My thirty-year-old brother is another story. He lives with my parents and has no life of his own. He has no friends, no job, and is very shy. I think because my mother couldn't fully control my sister and me, she focused on him. She has always told him what to do. Even now she treats him like a child. Before they leave the house, she asks him if he went to the bathroom. After all that overt protection, he now acts invisible. Even when he's there he's silent.

My illness has brought the two of us closer together. When I needed someone to drive me places my brother immediately offered to help. It was a good excuse for him to get away from my mother. Also, he was so happy that at last someone needed him. The first weekend Mark left, he came over to babysit so I could have some free time to myself. My illness makes him feel important to someone. Helping me gives him self-confidence, and he feels free with me. He can open up and talk. And I'm glad I can be there for him. Perhaps I'm not the only one to benefit from this illness.

In spite of all the positive things I've gained from my condition, sometimes I get mad, particularly when I see people walking or bicycling with their kids. Simple things. I used to love bicycling. Or when I see a beautiful, self-confident woman, I think, You don't know what can happen tomorrow. You never know.

I would never have imagined something like this could happen to me. But I never feel sorry for myself. I know the illness has actually served me. I can see that today. If not for the illness, I might have stayed with Mark because that's all I knew. The illness forced me to the edge, and the situation between Mark and me had to change. Today I feel very strong and self-confident. I have to live with the limitations of the illness, but I no longer have to live with the limitations others force upon me.

Today, I'm very clear on what I need and what I don't need. What I want and what I don't want. I'm more honest with myself and others. Before, I wasn't able to say no. I wanted people to like me. I didn't want to hurt anyone. Now I see that if I'm honest, they'll like me even more. But now I'm much more discriminating about the kind of people I want around me. I no longer see those who give me nothing. As a result, I have gained a few friends and have lost a few.

There are things that are really no longer important to me. Before, I was horrified by the atrocities committed in various parts of the world. I gave them a good deal of emotional energy. Today, I can agree that all these wars are terrible, but they don't cause me pain. They're not here, in my house. If someone I know dies, that would touch me. People dying in a war in another part of the world doesn't touch me in the same way.

Before, I expressed my opinions without thinking. Now, I think and then talk. My mind seems to have become keener. My sense of smell and hearing have also changed. I can smell a vase of flowers in the next room. I couldn't do that before. Maybe I now have more time to pay attention. Most of the time I'm sitting here alone, and I enjoy that very much. I have time to listen to everything. After the kids leave, I sit here quietly and listen to the sound of silence. Or a half-hour before the kids arrive, I'll enjoy a few minutes of silence. It's very comforting, soothing. Silence is like a vibration. A small motor. A soft hum. A gentle breeze, very gentle.

If I have the strength to live my life with this illness, then I'll have the strength to face whatever comes. I know my disease is just going to get worse and worse. I'm afraid that one day I won't be able to talk, either, and that's the only way I can express myself now. Three years ago, I said, "I'm afraid I'm going to lose my legs." Then I lost them and I said, "I can live with that."

The next step is the voice. Most people with this disease end up having problems with their speech. But I might die before that happens.

The actual act of dying will be reassuring. I will know this job is done. It's time for the next one. In each life we learn something different. And when a life is over, we have learned everything we needed to learn this time around. Before, I was afraid to die because I thought I would miss the ones I love. Now, I believe I will have my eyes on them after my life is over.

When I will be told I only have a week left to live, I'd like my daughters to put their beds beside mine and be with me twenty-four hours a day. I'd like them beside me when I'm dying because they're the most important people in my life, and they have given me the strength to live with this disease. Also, if they're with me they won't be afraid of death, and they'll be able to say, "I was with my mother till the very end."

A friend did that with her father when she was thirty. Her father, who had cancer, went home to die. She stayed with him twenty-four hours a day for a full month. One night she slept with him, one night her mother slept with him. She said during that month they told each other everything that needed to be said. After he died, she felt that having been with him till the very end was the most beautiful thing she had done in her life.

When I'm dead I want red roses put in my coffin and then I want to be cremated. I'm always cold. In the fire I'll finally be warm and comfortable. And I will be cremated surrounded by red roses, which to me symbolize love and beauty.

I believe we find a cure and get well on the other side of life. For me there is no hell on the other side. Everyone lives their own particular hell here on earth. Death will be a relief. Like in my dreams, I will be able to use my arms and legs again. And after I die it will be like a new start.

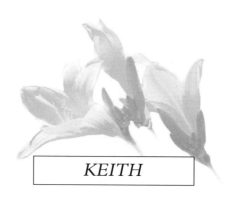

KEITH

Keith's name was given to me by the AIDS Society as someone who wanted and needed to talk. He was forty-six years old and had been a makeup artist in feature films, and having worked in films myself, I immediately knew what that world entailed. If you worked in films, you were judged by how you looked, presented yourself. I viscerally understood what he must have been up against with this disease.

I also understood that it was easy for someone in the film world to relate to his story as if it were a film script, as if it were someone else's story, which is exactly how our first three interviews transpired.

Admittedly, his story was a good one, but the stage directions for the lead actor — himself — were missing. He did not express the main character's emotional reactions. His wiry, nervous good looks conveyed only nonchalance. What were the emotions between the lines? Of course, I could fill them in without being told, but I wanted to know them from him. I kept asking how he felt when certain events happened. He was very casual in his response, while I was torn apart inside. I felt that the events he narrated and his emotions were very far apart, but I also felt that he very much wanted to talk.

After the third interview, I became frustrated. He had driven me home on his way to pick something up. In the car, once he had already arrived at my house, I took a deep, impatient breath and told him I had no sense of how the events he was relating had effected him emotionally. They sounded terrible, but he was talking about them in the most off-hand manner. I wanted his own emotional context. I did not want to fill it in myself. He listened, thinking, staring out the window. When I finished, he said his therapist had told him he was out of touch with his emotions. He told me he had taken primal therapy, and while two people were going hysterical beside him, punching the mats they lay on, he was thinking how lucky they were to be able to let go of all that. But he could not do it. He didn't even shed a tear.

At the next interview, I became more aggressive, asking him how he felt about certain events more and more often, insisting that he think about it now, in front of me. I approached the same question from many angles till he finally came up with an answer, till he could finally describe the feelings.

I want to slide into this illness, accept it, let it be. I don't want to see it as a tragic thing. But every new stage is a brand new experience, and I have no point of reference. A part of me is observing myself, like watching a movie, and it's a tearjerker. You get thinner, weaker, feverish, nauseous. Walking up the stairs is a little more difficult. Getting through the day is a little more tiring. Paul, a friend who lived upstairs, passed away from AIDS last year. When he was having trouble going up the stairs, I remember saying to myself, "I'm not going to let that happen to me." And it's happening.

I've cut out some of the pills because I couldn't afford them and they weren't helping me anymore. Certain pills make me nauseous or speedy. I sometimes get hypersensitive to smells, like cheap french fries. Just on a physical level, everyone reacts very differently. But I'm certain it's also connected to the psyche.

A part of me says, "I don't want to be sick, I want to be normal." Another part says, "It's okay, you can die. It'll be so peaceful when you finally rest." I'm looking forward to it. I don't have to do anything, as lazy as that sounds. I can simply let it happen. I see death as a liberation from this earthly body and these everyday things that can be hell.

I get anxious because I have to clear out a lot of my stuff, get rid of it before I die, and I don't have the discipline to organize myself. Then I decide I want to have my living room painted. Do I need to have it painted? Certainly not. But I hire these two guys at $160 a day to come in and paint. And I'm going to have the floor sanded. Why? Partly to keep things moving, to do something. But I should be concentrating on other things, like getting ready to go. Instead, I'm doing this. Maybe I want to see that room bright and beautiful. Maybe I'll move my bedroom in there. But this isn't really practical or useful. I think I need to do things that take me away from this illness.

You can't allow this AIDS thing to surround you constantly. I hate just running to the clinic, the pharmacy, the hospital, and the support group meetings. It's AIDS city. Talk to me about a new recipe or a new movie you saw. I want to be involved in life for as long as I can. It's up to me to keep myself busy, to keep my morale in top shape as much as possible, function as normally as possible. Live on a daily basis, do what I like to do in the couple of months or weeks I have left.

I have very little anxiety about time. Time is not my concern. When I will no longer have the energy to do what I want, I will be anxious to go. Some people go through months and months of suffering and boredom. Some just pray to die. A cousin died of bone cancer, and she suffered every day. For her, death was a form of grace. Why is the medical profession spending all this money to keep people alive? Take that money and use it for research. It's not going to help me to stay prostrate on a bed for another week or month or six months. Maybe people who are afraid to die want to hang on to every minute. I guess you never know what's coming, you only know when you're there. Who knows how I'll be when I get to that point? In the meantime I'm trying to do some work on myself.

I want to confront my immature and irrational feelings in time of panic. I must remember that a theme I should be working on is not to leave this life bitter or angry, in spite of the problems that arise. The last time I landed in emergency, I blew up at a fat little male nurse. Everything he did was wrong. I'm lying in bed with no water, nothing to pee in, and have to make a couple of phone calls because I've been there for twelve hours and you have to let people know where you are. Every time I asked him for something, he said, "That's not my job."

Finally, I blew up at him. How can I get what I want and be treated with respect without having to blow up? There is always some stupid complication, and I get so angry. Why is this happening to me? Then I catch myself and say, Don't play that game. I'm trying to deal with my anger in therapy right now.

Maybe part of my anger is that mine has not been a fully realized life. Being gay was the easiest route. My father used to say, "Go out and pinch the girls' asses. Grab their tits."

And I felt extremely anxious with women. I needed a woman to give me strength. I wanted someone to hold me in her arms. But I didn't know how to ask for that. My mother was not that physical. She was no Sophia Loren, and subsequently I'm attracted to women who are like goddesses, like my grandmother, with her perfume, her flowered dress, her ornate brooch. My grandmother was a busty thing with a heavy, corseted hip. I loved to be in her arms. I've never been into little girls and perky tits.

I clearly remember this actress from a few years ago. There was something goddess-like about her, and at the same time she was very vulnerable. I was an assistant makeup artist on this film, and one day she came to work after a hard night. She said to the makeup man, who was tall and elegant, "Oh, I need a hug."

He put his long, slender arms around her and just tapped her a few times on the back. I thought, "That's not what she wants. She needs a real hug." She was like a child, a vulnerable thing needing warmth from someone who wasn't going to judge her. When filming was over, we had a cast party. She was a little drunk, and we all had a good time with lots of champagne. I was very aware of her throughout the night. After the party, I asked her to come home with me, and she said, in a really shocked way, "Keith!"

She thought I was just with men. So it happened that night, shooting stars and waves crashing on the rocks. It lasted for a few weeks.

CR

The last heterosexual affair I had was with a stocky, chubby Jewish producer. Blond, lipliner, lip gloss, a ballsy kind of woman, but very sensual. I was turned on by her. And she was the most responsive ever. It was unbelievable. She was the first female who responded verbally to us in bed together. Others just giggled. Wendy said, "Oh, it feels good, I love what you do." It was marvellous.

I realized then that in another life I could get into this. Then it was, Come and meet my parents. And I ran away, because the more I was getting into it emotionally, the more anxious I was. I didn't have a clue how to deal with the anxiety.

I was vulnerable with women. My mother made me feel unsafe, she wasn't there to protect me from my father. She didn't have any strength to give me. At times I wasn't any more comfortable with men than with women. It was just easier. I could be aggressive with men. I didn't care. I simply told them to leave me alone if I had had enough.

I had fooled around with guys all through high school. But you never let on. I grew up in Shannon, a small Irish community north of Quebec City, where it was taboo to be a fifi. The guy I fooled around with had a girlfriend. But emotionally I just couldn't handle girls. As a teenager, I sat in the basement with this girl I thought was great. And I just wanted to be comfortable. I didn't want that edge. But I didn't know what to do, how to be. I wasn't going to get aggressive sexually. And I was paralyzed with anxiety, sitting next to her in the basement.

In high school I sat there thinking, Is someone going to come and rescue me? Of course, no one ever did. I could cry when I think that all I needed was five minutes of one person's time. It makes me angry that no one had the sensitivity to pay attention. I needn't have wasted so much time in anxiety. I could have gotten on with my life, been more efficient. All it would have taken was a word from my grandfather or uncle. Just a little pat on the shoulder, "Don't worry, you make a decision about what makes you happy, and respect yourself. You're part of our family, and we love you."

I needed that so much as I was growing up. I was suffering all the time. I hated school. I hated studying. I was uncomfortable with other people. I was not like them. I liked reading, painting, doing dolls' hair. Hair was my big escape. I was a freak kid who did dolls' hair. I couldn't get anyone to sit for me on a regular basis so I stole my sister's dolls and did their hair. They didn't talk back. I did these bouffant hairdos on them and had a great time.

To cope with the family dynamic, I built a fantasy world. I lived my most intense moments in my head, where I let out my anger and told people how I felt. The fun times were also lived in my head. I went shopping for clothes. I went dancing. All in my head. But there was always enough of me in the real world to maintain contact and function. I got dressed. I went to school on time. From the outside everything was normal. But it wasn't me.

About ten years ago, after I finished my primal therapy, I had a dream. My mother and I are in the dining room, and I hear my father coming. I become extremely anxious. I have never felt this anxious before in my whole life. My father is just about to enter the room, and I'm so overwhelmed by anxiety that the only recourse I have is to just go mad. I throw myself on the floor and yell from the pit of my being. My mother is not reacting because she knows I'm not mad. That was my way of hanging on. Hanging on in the face of pain by escaping into myself. So I still existed in reality, though I was not fully in it.

From a young age, my father always made me feel inadequate because I hadn't noticed this or that, or hadn't felt this or that. He often said, "You don't know what it's like. You'll never know."

Once, after having taken Aunt Vera to visit Uncle Stuart at the old folks' home, he described her leaning over to give Stuart a goodbye kiss. To hear my father say it, it was the most tender kiss anybody could have ever given anybody. It touched him profoundly and was a thing of immense beauty for him. But he made you feel you could never be his equal because you hadn't seen it, you weren't there, or what do you know, anyway?

When I was ten, he wanted to show me how to shovel snow. Not only did he do it better because he was an adult and more coordinated, but he doubled his energy and did it like a madman. There was no hope of keeping up with him. I wasn't even going to try because I didn't want the anxiety. I remember thinking, I couldn't do anything, or accomplish anything, or finish anything. I became this sensitive freak.

Strangely enough, I probably inherited this sensitivity from my father. He was diagnosed as a mild paranoid schizophrenic, and there were all sorts of situations that set him off.

From the time I can remember, after a crisis, my father would sit me down opposite him at the kitchen table, and he would drink, talk to me, and sob. He told me stories of his past and cry and cry and cry about how he loved his father and his father was mean to him. He was extremely intense. By the time he was twenty-six, he had seven-eighths of his stomach removed because he was full of ulcers.

My father came from a strange background. He didn't talk about it in detail, but when he was six years old, he caught his mother with the butcher, and he was shattered. The mother probably never got any affection or love from her husband and gave herself to the first person who paid her attention. He was the oldest of three boys, and there had also been a half-sister from the mother's side who had committed suicide, and he took the world on his shoulders. His father was so unhappy, either because his wife had all these affairs or he lost his money in the stock market or he was just a miserable son of a bitch. He regularly pushed his oldest son around or came home after work and beat him up. He took his frustration out on the kids and his wife. And my father had to leave school to work and put food on the table.

As he told me stories about his past at the kitchen table, I sat there and cried with him. I was the only one he could talk to, who listened to him. The man was highly sensitive and had nowhere to turn. It must have been very lonely to have all these feelings of shame about his own family. When he went to see the psychiatrist, he was just pumped full of pills and couldn't get it up anymore.

Much later, I realized that I had developed a guilt complex about my father's youth. I felt responsible for his unhappiness.

CB

He came from Detroit to Quebec City looking for work and met my mother's family. Irish, good-hearted, hard-working, salt-of-the-earth farmers. They were very family-oriented, with cousins and aunts and my grandparents, with the country house and the city house that was the social hub for the whole family. My father walked into this scenario, the warm family, the togetherness, and was overwhelmed. He fell in love with the beautiful eldest daughter and was on his best behaviour.

My father was Mr. Nice Guy before my mother married him. After the marriage, he began criticizing everything. She didn't know how to handle him. She was not confrontational, not expressive. She was timid. When he went into his crisis mode and cried to me about his family, he also put her family down. My drunk father said, "Why don't you tell your son about your father, the homosexual?"

Inside I thought, "Hey, that's great news, I'm not alone."

Apparently my grandmother saw my grandfather, fully clothed, push up against Mr. Andrew's butt. But my family is crazy, we'd goof around, play sexually. Maybe my grandfather was just playing around that split second she was standing at the doorway. But it became a family scandal and a hidden secret. And my father would use this against my mother.

My mother and father were not exactly a match made in heaven. Sex was tremendously important for my father. And my mother didn't have a natural desire or curiosity, whereas her younger sister, my aunt, liked men, and she was a frisky little pony. I always thought that was a gift. I don't want to put my mother down, but she just never had that gift. My father had it, along with a tremendous need to be loved physically. I can imagine his one-way street with my mother. I'm sure he knew that she loved him, but not in a lusty way, like, Come here, baby, Mama can take care of you. That's what I always wanted in a woman when I was a teenager.

My mother just treated me like poor little Keith, your father is so hard on you. And she used me to whine about my father. My grandmother was not a very open-minded woman and would not have been very sympathetic to my mother's complaints about him. Her attitude was, That's the man you married, and that's the man you stay with. He brings home his pay.

She also needed someone to talk to, and I was all she had. I know she appreciated my listening to her. But I didn't like the feeling of her confiding in me. It made me very uncomfortable. My hatred for my father was easy to manifest. I could tell him I hated him. But I didn't realize I felt any negativity toward my mother. Years later, when I did my primal, I saw she was as responsible for my anxiety as he was, and all this anger toward her came out. I just let her use me.

I felt sorry for my mother. One time, when I was already an adult, my father said, "Oh, I never hit your mother." When I heard this I was furious. Of course he hit her. I remember going somewhere in the car, and he leaned over and just smashed her in the face with the back of the hand. And he says to my face, "I have never hit your mother."

He didn't hit her that often, but with age it escalated. You'd think by the time she's in her menopause and he's heading for retirement things would be a little easier. You don't have to go into a crisis mode every few months. But when he's fifty-six years old, he bangs her around and rips her pyjamas off. That was it. I said to my mother, "You do what you want, but if you stay in the house with him, I'm never coming back to visit."

We all threw that ultimatum at her, and that's when she left. She asked me to testify in court on her behalf. I said, "Sure."

He was very upset with me. She needed my support. I'm not going to support him.

But there were some very nice things too. One day, when I was about fifteen, I found a place that had the top-of-the-line French curling irons, and I wanted one. I asked my parents for it. One day my father drove me into town and handed me a blank check for the curling iron. I was thrilled. That was the summer I lost my virginity with a girlfriend and then became infested with crabs.

Also, my father did home movies of us as kids, and watching them today, I can see he loved us dearly. The man had such a huge love to give. He just didn't know how. As the first son, I think he loved me too much, and that's what scared me about him. Once, when I was about ten, he said to me, I loved you so much as a baby I would have eaten the shit out of your diapers. And I just thought, Yech. How can a kid relate to that?

Maybe he thought his love for his family was going to take away his demons, but they didn't. In all his madness, he was fucking lonely. He had no buddy. The Irish have no imagination, they didn't accept someone who was a little different, emotionally intense. The ones who were more sensitive took to the bottle to ease their tension, and that was accepted. My father was not a bad man. He brought his paycheque home. We were always clean, dressed, well fed. And there were many simple little things. At the end of a meal, my father would say, "I've had an elegant sufficiency." He put his fork and knife on the plate, and that was the sign that the meal was over. And I've always done that.

He also had a poetic side to him that's absolutely thrilling. After my parents separated he got an apartment in Lachine that I described as a schizophrenic's apartment. He made a lamp with a pie plate, painted his face on it, poked holes all around and put pigeon feathers through the holes. It was magnificent, not the kind of thing I'd want in here, but it had tremendous impact. And my father was a self-taught draftsman. He did structural steel drawings, all accompanied by impeccably printed notes. And he had beautiful pens and rulers. He worked at Dominion Bridge where he was promoted to chief draftsman and had over a dozen men under him. But my father has absolutely no taste. He'll go into a department store and think he's getting the greatest bargain and buy the cheapest polyester suit. Tacky shoes and a tacky shirt. He has no sense of quality. He just loves the gaudy stuff.

Maybe, in some strange way, my father had an influence on the direction my life took, my interest in hair and makeup. Perhaps it was a reaction to his gaudiness, or maybe I inherited his creativity.

After high school I didn't know who I was and where I was going. I took a hairdressing course and went to work in a salon as an assistant. There was another assistant, a girl, who took a shine to me and seduced me. We went out for a while, but I had the hots for the hairdresser I was assisting. One day I wrote him a note saying I wanted to have an affair. He read the note right in the staff room and said, "Well, what time should we meet on Sunday?" I had to sit down, I was blown away.

Having both a girlfriend and boyfriend brought up such guilt. I had this vision of meeting God on Judgement Day and being told, You just had to be a little more courageous and you could have been straight and you wouldn't have had this problem of sexuality.

I thought maybe I had been lazy about it, maybe I hadn't worked hard enough to go toward a straight relationship. But that was my way of remaining sane in this life. I didn't want to freak out anymore. I didn't want the anxiety. I just wanted to live. To escape the confusion, I went to British Columbia.

On Friday I got off the train in Vancouver and went straight to the top salon in the country. By Tuesday I was working there as shampoo boy, blow dryer, learn as you go. Within a month I became one of the top assistants. Frans, the best hairdresser in the salon, was like a god, a mysterious poet. He was an artist at doing hair, weighing texture, shape, balance, light. I thought he was brilliant. Subtle, not flamboyant, fluffy, obvious stuff. He had such style, and I was attracted to him. We did speed one night and stayed up talking about life and art.

At this point I was sharing an apartment with two English hairdressers. Frans was not getting along with his wife. One night he called and said, "Can I come over? I can't stay here anymore."

I said, "Fine."

During that night, he made a move on me. I couldn't believe it. I thought I had been touched by God. And we started an affair. Sex threw me off course. Or maybe it was the combination of sex and emotional involvement. I wasn't able to be in a relationship and remain objective about who I was relative to who that person was. I lost myself. If the sex was good, I was just blinded. I was in love. I couldn't think clearly. I forgot about what I wanted to do, the things that made me who I was, and totally gave myself over to the other person. I lost my personality.

I felt privileged to be in Frans's company. He saw things so differently from anyone else. We did a lot of marijuana together, and I was hypersensitive to grass. A joint blew me away for a day, whereas other people could do two or three a night. As I smoked, my palms began to sweat, my anxiety grew, and my demons started coming to the surface, demons I wasn't even aware were there. I had no control over the anxiety and didn't know how to express it. I sat there looking totally normal while inside I was dying.

When I wasn't smoking, I was in a daydream world. In my head, Frans and I talked about perfection, beauty, awareness. All this wonderful, idealistic stuff. I could clearly verbalize my thoughts. In my head was the room where I lived and talked to Frans, where everything was beautiful. We made love or went out to eat. It was all the way I wanted it to be. In my head was real life, where I fully lived and expressed my emotions. I was fully myself, the self I wanted to be.

There was a certain amount of realism to my external existence, otherwise I would have been in a mental institution. I found jokes funny. I told my own jokes. I had my preferred place for hamburgers. But life in my head was stronger, it had much more shape.

Frans stayed with me for a while in that room, and then he moved out. I was grief-stricken.

One night I had to speak to him. I took some LSD and went to his new flat where he lived alone. When I got there, he was out. I climbed in through the window and sat in the dark waiting for him. He came home and turned on the light. When he saw me, I was about to say something and nothing came out. But I had everything inside. He just looked at me as I sat there totally paralyzed. At that moment I ceased to exist.

That night was a turning point in my life. I realized I had been living in a dream for the last twenty years of my life. I didn't want to live in a fantasy world anymore. The fantasies couldn't be applied to real life. There was no connection between the two worlds. I was angry with myself. I wanted to be more aware and more efficient with my emotions. Either I was hyper or terribly lazy. I was frustrated with my hyper side and annoyed with my lazy side.

I decided to make a conscious effort to be more alert and would try to catch myself. Whenever my mind veered off reality, I'd say, "No fantasy, no imagination. No fantasy, no imagination." I'd repeat that all day long. Soon I was mumbling.

I went to see a psychiatrist and was put on tranquilizers. Then I became extremely depressed and really went crazy. I spent a few months in a psychiatric hospital, and when I got out I felt overwhelming guilt. So I started going to church. That didn't give me anything. Then I felt I had to discipline myself because I had never disciplined myself before in my life. I started jogging. I went out and ran full blast, without even warming up. My legs became swollen, and I had excruciating pain.

At this point, I couldn't take it anymore and had my first suicide attempt. Drank some toxic product at the salon. When I began to feel strange, I walked out the front door, took a taxi and said, "Take me to the hospital." And they pumped my stomach.

After my fourth suicide attempt, I said to myself, Come on, if you're ever going to do this, do it seriously or not at all. They were feeble cries for help. Now, I sometimes think, If I can get through this life without killing myself, I've accomplished something.

I couldn't stay in Vancouver anymore and went back to live with my parents. I looked terrible, skin and bones, hollow-eyed. What I look like now. Sharon, who was two years older, was no longer at home. But there was Debbie, Eddie, and Pamela, who were seven, eleven, and fourteen years younger than me. I was their weird older brother, and we had a great time together. I rediscovered my childhood. We played cowboys and Indians with the neighbourhood kids. I was the Indian chief. It was fun.

But I still felt guilty about having lived in a fantasy world. Felt guilty about all those years in my head, with Frans and me and my father and telling him to go to hell. None of that was real. I didn't exist. I had to get in touch with reality.

CR

One night I was walking in Quebec City and heard piano music. I followed the sound to a dance school with mirrors, barres, and people doing exercises. I inquired and registered for dance classes. Bought myself some tights, shoes, and a T-shirt and took nine classes a week for a year and a half. I was terrible, but I wasn't going to make a career out of it. Dance gave me self-confidence and changed my body, my posture. I wasn't pigeon-toed anymore. My spine straightened. I had a way of carrying myself. For the first time in my life, at the age of twenty-six, I finally found my body, connected with it in a physical way. I was reborn. There were no more extremes of very active and very lazy. The scenarios in my head lessened. And I stopped taking Valium. I became a whole person. As crazy as it sounds, dance humanized me. As I learned to live in the real world, there was less anxiety, less suffering. I was able to express anger, dissatisfaction. I could verbalize my feelings.

By now I was getting bored doing hair. When it finally dawned on me how to do hair efficiently and I learned to relax, like, you don't have to do the perfect haircut on every person, I started developing speed and became more creative. But then I didn't want to do it anymore. You can fall asleep in a salon on Tuesday afternoon at two-thirty. If I have nothing to do, I get anxious or tired. I hate waiting, and I hate being kept waiting.

I have a real thing about having to wait. Indirectly it has to do with the time my mother was pregnant with me. At the time, Sharon, who was two, needed a lot of attention. My father was very demanding, criticizing everything from the housecleaning to the food. My mother must have thought, What have I gotten myself into, marrying this maniac who isn't happy with anything and this squawking child? And she just resisted having me.

When I finally arrived, my sister always had to be fed first because she was screaming hysterically. I was told, "You were such a good baby, you never said a word." Exactly. In all my baby pictures, my sister is wildly grinning for the camera, and I look like I don't want to be here. The issue of waiting has been a real motif in my life.

Much later, when I worked long hours on films, my free time was precious. I didn't want to waste it waiting. And I always had to wait for Paul. I would say, "Don't keep doing this to me." He always did. I always bitched about it. He'd say, "Relax." I'd silently go mad. Paul was a professional student with lots of free time and was used to a certain pace. In spite of the waiting, I was always so happy to be with him. I took him to restaurants, bought him clothes, took him on trips.

But at this point, in Quebec City, I still hadn't met Paul.

Soon after I finished my dance classes, I got a job as an extra on a feature film. There was no hairdresser on set. The makeup person knew I was a hairdresser and some days called me in to help get the actors' hair ready. Whenever I could, I watched him do makeup and was fascinated.

My next move was to Montreal, to take a facial course for nine months. Here I was, twenty-eight, and I was in school again. I thought this was great. When my facial course ended, I called the makeup man I had worked with on the feature and asked if he needed someone. He said, "Can you come Tuesday?"

I showed up at the crack of dawn, a makeup assistant on a film, with a box of Kleenex, lipsticks, and the powder puff to touch people up. On set, I was surrounded by all these well-known personalities. And I was comfortable. I felt at home on a film shoot. I left hair behind and embarked upon a career as a makeup artist. I loved it. It appealed to the Gemini in me. The work was always different, challenging. Working on films gave me time off, allowed me to travel and meet all kinds of different people.

Frans used to say, "Life can be a poem, it can be extraordinary." Yes, life can be a poem. And some films have been poems to do with people who trust each other. A problem is openly discussed. There is no blame, no hurt feelings. It can happen. I have worked with classy actors, talented, intelligent people. And they respected me because I demanded respect. I expected them to be on time, not to be on the cellular phone or smoking while I'm doing makeup on them. This is our time, and this is for the character.

A successful career is about knowing what to say, how to say it, how to handle yourself and situations. I wasn't good at handling situations of a confrontational nature. I didn't know how to deal with authority. There was still a tremendous amount of anger inside.

Part of the imperfection in my relationship with Paul was my inability to express anger. He laughed at me in front of people once, and inside myself I thought, How can you do this, after everything I've done for you? When he asked me later what was wrong, I explained very reasonably. He just waved it away. And I couldn't show him the anger I felt, which made me even more angry inside. After he died, I gave it to him. I told him exactly how I felt. I yelled. Finally, I allowed myself to express the anger. It was liberating.

When it came to work, I was too outspoken. I didn't hold back enough. Vincent told me I had psychological problems. I have jumped into situations in a confrontational way because I was feeling stupid and insecure and had to defend myself. The film business can be very snotty, and you have to appear to know what you're doing even if you don't. There were times I didn't have exciting solutions for things. Sometimes they were mediocre. Maybe I was defensive at moments. But so were a lot of other people. With time, I became better and better. I evolved without being front-page news.

I'm proud of who I am. My brother and sisters were minor celebrities because of me. Everyone from Shannon was asking them, "What's Keith doing?" When I went for a visit everyone in town wanted to know what actor or actress I've been working with. That was fun and good for my ego.

This spring the word got out that I had AIDS. I knew if the people in the industry found out the phone would stop ringing for work. Now everyone knows about me. And I haven't gotten a call for a film in months, and there are films going on left and right. To be realistic, I wouldn't be able to do a feature now. You have to be in top shape to absorb that stress. Still, it would be nice to get a call, even for a few days' work. One company that does TV commercials still calls me.

Sometimes I ask myself why I'm doing makeup. Maybe because I love experimenting with colour. When I began going to museums, looking at paintings, I woke up to the possibilities of colour. The greens, blues, yellows, and ochres that Van Gogh used made his canvases vibrate. I'm quite uneducated in terms of art. I know your Gauguin and Monet, though I didn't get any of this at home. I got it from Vincent, who danced with the Metropolitan Opera and went to all the museums when he was on tour.

Vincent and I were an item for a year and a half, near the end of his dance career. I met him right after my facial course. He's a very well-read person, though he wasn't the best dancer in the world. He has always been very generous with his time and knowledge of art and films. He took the time to explain things.

I had a terrible complex about what I didn't know. I allowed myself to feel stupid. Vincent taught me to ask questions. As I became more and more a part of his circle, I became more confident. Vincent helped me to feel comfortable with people, even if I just sat there and didn't say a word. I knew things they didn't know, like film technique. As my film career developed, people became interested in what I did, and when it became a topic of conversation, my enthusiasm was infectious.

At one point, Vincent said, "Why don't you move in with me?" He had a beautiful apartment filled with books, antiques, a crystal chandelier in the dining room, very European. It was a magical place. I thought, I'm going to be swallowed up in his world. I need my own space.

Soon after our relationship ended, I met Paul. I met him at a disco where a group of us had gone dancing and Paul fainted. Me and another guy carried him down the stairs to help him get some fresh air. As we were walking down, I looked at him. He had this long, thick hair and burnished skin. He was so beautiful. The next time I saw him was in a gay bar. I'm standing there having a beer, and along comes Paul. He's surprised to see me here because when we first met I was with a woman. He buzzed around me. I buzzed around him for a while. And he invited me to his place. That began a weekend of passion. I was immensely attracted to him and immediately in love. This was the most exotic and sensual creature you could ever imagine. He wasn't masculine and he wasn't feminine, just utterly sensual. I was overwhelmed. I was in awe of him, the way he moved, the way he thought, the way he dressed, the Lebanese food he ate. I was in love with absolutely everything he did. He had stuffed animals on his bed, and I felt so safe in his place. I'd go there when I was anxious and would sleep like a god. I always felt safe in Paul's surroundings.

He was the only person in my life I just loved. He evoked the most complete emotions in me. I felt paternal, maternal, brotherly toward him. And there was passion. There was everything. And Paul had a terrific sense of humour. He could have me in stitches. We could be totally silly together. And my family loved him. He was invited to all the family events, made us all laugh.

There was something innocent and childlike about him. He was in another world. He never worried about money, and it always showed up, thanks to me or his mother or whoever else. We went through a period of smoking coke, and he smoked the most in our group but never bought any. Everyone offered him theirs. He never had any worries. He never wanted for anything. If he needed a pair of jeans, I'd say, "I'll get them for you." And off we went. In Provincetown, I bought him shoes, a leather jacket. Half my money was spent on stuff for him. It was my pleasure to do it. I know I bought his affections. It was one means I had that other people in his life didn't.

The relationship never developed romantically. He had just come out of a very heavy relationship where his boyfriend beat him up. This was his first boyfriend after he left his mother's house at seventeen. When I met him, he was nineteen and I knew this kid had a lot more living to do. I didn't have what it took to really keep his attention for the rest of my life. It was like having an extraordinary bird presented to you, and you either try to keep it in a cage or you just let it go, hoping it will come back. And he kept coming back to me as a friend, and he kept coming back more and more. Then he started doing work on himself and discovered his anger at his father. He saw that a lot of people around him were taking pieces of him.

He said, "You're the only one who doesn't want a piece of me, and I can talk to you." I was totally flattered by this. I was becoming Paul's best friend. He respected me and confided in me. I was honoured by efforts he made to come into my world, to know my weak points and smooth them over.

When I was thirty-eight, soon after Paul had begun his sessions with a psychologist, I started primal therapy, and we began to open up to each other. Paul was the person who knew the most about me.

I got to primal through a friend who lent me *The Primal Scream* by Arthur Janov. I couldn't put it down after the first paragraph. At this point I was coping with my life better than I ever had. But the book helped me see inside. I thought, Maybe I should deal with the pain just to make myself more efficient emotionally. I went to therapy for a year, and a half with fourteen other people and two therapists.

During the sessions, people were opening like popcorn. The pain they were able to release was unbelievable. They wailed, cried, screamed. The amount of emotion expressed in that room was scary. I just lay there on my mat. I couldn't open my mouth. The therapist said I was very resistant. In my head I kept thinking, I'm like a firecracker. But I can't afford to be humiliated. Then there were only two of us left in the group, a girl and me. I had my back to her, and she was wailing and wailing. I envied her. I couldn't even groan. Then, finally, I just exploded. I discovered that I had this tremendous anger for my mother. I thought it was going to be a Dad theme and it was a Mom theme. Surprise!

After that, I was able to express my anger to her for not controlling the situation with my father. Once I said, "Why didn't you take the plate of potatoes and bash him on the head when he was being a little prick at the dinner table?" That's when it dawned on me why I was angry with her. She played the victim all those years with my father. My mother said, "Well, you couldn't divorce your husband at that time, and I stayed with him because of you kids." Look, there's been women before you and since and there will always be women who have taken their destiny into their own hands. You have to stand up and take your place at one point. But my mother had to pay attention to society.

Even from the time she left my father, she played the victim. She went to live with her brother in Quebec City and was like a lost child. I said, "You can get a job as a doctor's receptionist. You have to dress up in an office, and it'll be good for you."

"No, no."

"There's a whole world that can open up to you. You can have a great time. Take a little secretarial course in the evenings. Your life is yours." She was in her fifties, able-bodied and bilingual.

"No, no." She went to work at Sears for the switchboard, just what she had done when she married my father, and never evolved beyond that. She was not an adventurous person, not the kind to take a situation in hand and make something of it. And I needed that. I told her, "I need you to give me some strength. I need you to give me something. You've got to leave me with something."

I know my criticism hurt her. But I had to hurt her. My anger made her very sad. She'd say, "In my day . . ."

"Fuck your day, we're in the nineties and so much progress has been made. People are asking themselves questions today. I don't want to hear about your time anymore. You're an intelligent, grown-up woman. You can change your thinking. Open your eyes. Think for yourself."

Maybe she didn't totally understand me, but fifteen years after she had been separated from my father, she allowed herself to get angry at him. She'd say, "Every time I think of that son of a bitch, all those years . . ." She'd sit there and cry.

I thought, "Finally." And we were able to be friends.

I think I loved her more when I became capable of accepting her weaknesses, her limits. Although I would have wished it to be otherwise, and I was angry about it, she was doing what she needed to do to keep herself together at the time.

Four years ago, she got emphysema and had trouble getting around. I took her places and picked things up for her. I did what I could. She was in and out of the hospital for tests. And her condition was getting worse. The doctor wanted her to go into hospital twice a week for an exercise program.

I said, "That's it, you're moving in with me. When I can, I'll drive you down to the clinic, and when I can't you'll take a taxi. I'm going to take care of you." It came from the heart. This is my mother, and I've got to help her.

A week later, she was gasping for breath and had to be admitted to hospital.

We all knew this was the last stretch. Whenever she'd bring up death, I'd say, "Well, how does that make you feel?" I encouraged her to express herself. I wanted to help her die. Physically she didn't suffer, but she was afraid. I told her, "It's fine, when the time comes just let yourself go. Let it be easy."

Five days later she hemorrhaged internally. I held her arm as she was going and said, "It's okay, don't be afraid, let yourself go." I caressed her hand, and she just slipped away. It was sad but beautiful, peaceful. After resenting my mother throughout my childhood because I was her ear and then expressing my anger towards her, it was a privilege to share that last moment with her.

Now, at the age of forty-seven, part of me is fighting off feeling guilty that if my father has to die in the gutter, then so be it. I don't want to feel guilty, I don't give a shit what happened to you, I'm sorry it happened, but I wasn't there, and it's not my fault. You deal with it.

I know he loves me, and I love him, but we have absolutely nothing to say to each other. I see him once a year at Christmas, and that's it. I give him a big hug and he gives me a big hug and we wish each other Merry Christmas. If we speak, we argue. It's been like this since he moved out of here three years ago.

He was living in Quebec City and one day called me to announce he was moving. By now my mother was dead. The next thing I know, he is in Montreal with his truck and all his furniture. He calls to say, "I've got a few things here, can I put them in your place for a while?"

"Sure."

He knew my front room was empty because, by now, my brother and his wife had moved out. Three days later he's moved in. It happened so quickly. He doesn't ask me. Doesn't sit me down, we should have a talk, this is what I'm thinking of doing, would you mind, can we make an arrangement. Nothing. Nada. And I'm in a dilemma. He's my father. I want to help. But at the same time, I deserve respect. Tell me what your intentions are. How long are you thinking of staying? I have to go to him and ask, "What's going on?"

He stands there beating around the bush. Much later, I said, "You drive me crazy, you sit around all day, watching TV, smoking cigarettes, doing nothing. Go do some volunteer work. Take painting classes." For over a year, he sits there and looks out the window.

One night we have a party upstairs, at Paul's. We finish at five in the morning. I say to a good friend of mine, "It's crazy to go home, come and sleep at my place, I have a big bed."

The next morning, the two of us are sleeping in bed, naked, and the door is open a crack because of the cat. I hear my father get up, walk down the hall, and stop adjacent to my room. He spends about seven minutes in front of my door, looking in. Then he calls Paul's mother to tell her he's caught the two of us in bed together. What has he seen? Two people sleeping in a bed, and it's not even Paul.

Had Paul's mother not known he was gay, he could have created a scandal. As far as she's concerned I'm like a brother to Paul. And she just laughed at him. I could have slapped him. You have no business putting your nose in my private life. After that I told him to leave. I don't care where you go, just go. Out. And he left without a word. Without an apology.

The whole time he was here, I never told him I was HIV positive. He doesn't know I have AIDS now, and I don't want him to know. He's a stupid man who doesn't know how to handle it. He can't be trusted.

CB

By the time I got AIDS, Paul had passed away. I thought I would die before him because he ran around less than I did, and we were both diagnosed HIV positive around the same time. When Paul got sick, I was working on a TV series which lasted through his illness and death. It's only now that I feel I've made some progress with the mourning. At the time, I couldn't cry. I was numb. I had lost my child, my lover, my best friend. Paul was everything to me.

A few weeks ago, in a meditation class, we were told to visualize ourselves in a comfortable, safe place. I visualized Paul's room. He was sleeping curled up in his bed. I kissed him on his forehead, his nose, anywhere and everywhere. It was not sexual. It was just love, a love that encompasses everything. Sexuality, sensuality, tenderness. It was very peaceful. Kissing him all over was the beginning of the mourning process. Now I tell him I love him all the time. Sometimes I conjure up his image as I saw him in the meditation class and gently kiss him and hold him just to soothe myself.

Kissing Paul all over is about allowing myself to totally express my love for him with no holds barred. When he was alive, I didn't let him know what my real feelings were because it would have made him uncomfortable and it could have ruined the relationship. But all he would have had to say was, We're together, and I would have dropped everything. I would have been devoted to him.

The last time I conjured up his image, I heard myself saying in my head, I love you but I want you to love me, too. I want you to want to be with me as much as I want to be with you. For me, he was the one. But was I the one for him? I had the impression that I loved him more than he loved me. Maybe I had limitations as far as he was concerned.

Paul didn't give a lot of affection until the last two years of his life. Then he would attack me and tickle me. And I thought, Isn't that funny, he can't just say, I like you or love you and give me a big hug. It was a very adolescent way for him to express affection, but I accepted it. It was his way of getting close to me physically. After a tussle, we'd roll around on the floor and laugh.

When he was dying, a part of me was jealous because he always had Miles, his boyfriend, and his mother around his bed, and the two

were fighting for his attention. His mother was constantly fawn-
ing over him. From the moment that child was born, she was an
overpowering, overwhelming presence. When the father left she
overprotected him. He was this spoiled child who always got his way.
The two manipulated each other to the day he died.

AIDS changes you. Toward the end, Paul panicked, and he became
very selfish, very demanding. He ordered Miles and his mother
around. They did whatever he wanted. His mother would have been
willing to lie down in front of a transport truck if it was going to help
her son. She didn't have much money, and some of Paul's medication
was very expensive. His attitude was, I'm your son. How can you
think of money when I'm dying?

Part of his problem was that he had all this time to think about his
illness, to ponder it. He was doing his master's in anthropology. He
didn't have a care in the world, he was getting loans and bursaries,
and he had no ambition beyond that. When he got sick, he stopped
going to school and was running from one doctor's appointment to
another, taking everything and anything. And that's not what I would
have expected of him. Before Paul got sick, I thought he had a strong
philosophy of life. This was the most natural person I had ever met
who fascinated me. And he didn't end up that way.

As he got sick, he became slower and slower. I was always waiting
for him. The day before my mother's funeral, he and I shared a room
at the Hilton. The next morning, he got up before seven, ordered
coffee from room service, and sat gazing out the picture window. I
said, "Come on, we have to go."

"Don't rush me."

I felt like hitting him over the head, Paul, this is not your day to
say this, it's my mother's funeral. I'm not going to be late because
you are lost in thought! But I didn't say anything.

After the funeral, we went to have a Chinese buffet, and my father
showed everyone a picture of my mother and me which had been
taken when she visited me on a film set. This was taken after the two
had already divorced. And someone had folded me out of the
picture. When I saw it, I was so insulted. Not only does he have it,
but I'm folded out of it. I said, "Where did you get that?"

He said nothing. My father is so sneaky. After my mother left him, he used to harass her regularly, following her around in his car. She was terrified of him.

I wish I could have given her security. It's sad to think that you can't give someone eternal security. I was thinking today, There's nothing permanent, everything is always changing. It would be nice to say evolving.

But I do believe in love. In my idealistic state, I believe we're all meant to love each other. I have tried to put it into practice. Just loving a person and accepting them for who they are is a big feat. A relationship is probably the most important work we'll do on this earth.

I think one of my goals here on earth is to help my brother, to encourage him, tell him he's smart, a wonderful person. I try to give him something. I remember my mother saying, "Oh, your brother, he's never going to amount to much."

How can you say that about your own son? My brother's best gift is a childlike innocence. He just glowed when he was young. We used to call him Sunshine. When he was thirteen, my father had yet another crisis and ended up in hospital. The doctors pumped him full of drugs till he turned into a vegetable. Eddie didn't have anybody. The kid took a dive and ended up in hospital himself. He lost all his sense of security, all his self-confidence. From that point on, he closed. But I relate to that boy inside. I know you're scared because you're sensitive. That sensitivity is a gift from God, don't ever be ashamed of it. Turn it into your strength, instead of seeing it as a weakness. Make an effort to be positive. Have the confidence to do what you want. Make yourself happy. But he conforms. He wants to keep the peace, and that adds pressure to an already stressful life of being a father, making mortgage payments, doing shift work. By sixty he'll be worn right down by life. All because he's afraid.

If you don't allow yourself to be afraid, life can be a poem. Life can be a poem if you work at it, work on yourself, look inside, look outside. Man's nature is to ascend. It doesn't have to be every moment or every day. As long as you're working on the ascension, you can be more sensitive and tender in the love you give. Perhaps this is the time to return to the conversations in my head, to nurture and strengthen my idealism. It might alleviate the anger, the anxiety. And I'll be able to slide into death from a fullness.

But I'm left with my hunger for the love that's all encompassing. Paul came close though I couldn't abandon myself to it totally. Love is a gift that takes courage and work. Then there can be intense happiness and extraordinary love, where it's passion, comfort, and trust, all those things in a trashy, romantic novel. The love that takes you over the top, and you explode and never come back to earth because you don't need to. One day, in another life, I'll find that all-encompassing love.

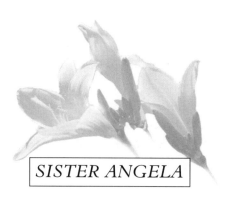

I had spent considerable time looking for a nun, priest, or rabbi to interview, anyone who represented religious faith, any faith. I thought that those who had spent most of their lives communing with God, praying in their fashion, being in touch with more esoteric concerns than day-to-day life must have a special insight into death. I had heard about a rabbi with a brain tumour, but he refused to talk to me.

I continued my search. Finally I heard about Sister Angela, a seventy-eight-year-old nun who had been the Mother Superior of her convent. She was dying of cancer. When I contacted her, she sounded weak but very willing to help. But she was not certain if she was strong enough to talk for more than one hour at a time.

She was in a church hospital with other nuns, though she had a spacious private room. At the foot of her bed was a table with two chairs. This is where we talked. She wore a grey A-line skirt with a white tailored shirt and a grey cardigan. A nurse took me into her room, where she welcomed me with a friendly smile.

As the first interview progressed, I could tell this was an adventure for her. She was more than willing to revisit memories, look once more at how certain events had transpired in her life, why she had done certain things. She welcomed talking about the people who had passed through her life. And I was curious about what a nun's life was like. I was surprised to learn that the difficulties in her life were similar to those we all face.

The interviews, which actually lasted closer to two hours, were very tiring for her. I was grateful for the time she had given me and appreciated her warning. It gave me time to prepare, to decide which questions were the most important.

I've been in this infirmary one year and four months. I'm here to stay for the rest of my days, with nothing more to do but prepare for eternity. Though my time has come and my days of teaching are over, my life has not yet ended. To my surprise, I'm still learning and growing. Obviously, God still has plans for me, even though I'm now virtually immobile. This illness is giving me the time and opportunity to get to know myself better, in a way I have not yet done while serving Him. Whatever happens is God telling us to wake up and pay attention. The time has come for me to live the advice He has helped me give to others.

I began to think of death in a more concrete way about five years ago, when I was invited to help our elderly sisters who were sick and dying. I took care of them, talked to them, comforted them. Very often they said, "I'm useless now. I can do nothing in this condition." I touched their arm or shoulder and gently said, "This is not the time to do. You have already done everything you could. Now you are allowed to simply be."

Since quite a few were afraid of dying, I didn't want to aggravate their fear by talking about death. Instead, we spoke about life. I asked them why they had joined the order and what they had learned by living in the community. I told them that, in looking over their life, God was preparing them for the end of their journey on earth. As we talked, I myself started to examine death and, I suppose, began to prepare myself in a rather abstract way.

At the time, I considered the sisters who were sick and dying to be old. Then I was seventy-three and, in comparison, I thought of myself as young. I was their hands and their eyes. I wrote their letters. I got them whatever they needed. I was agile, energetic. Today I'm seventy-eight, and in the last five years, physically, I've grown old. I have a good friend who is ninety-two, and both in looks and spirit I consider her much younger than myself. I hardly have the energy to walk around my room. Now I'm the one who relies on others for help.

My present problem started fourteen years ago with a very atypical form of tuberculosis. The doctors found a hole at the top of my lungs, and one-third of my lungs had to be removed. Now I only have two-thirds left to breathe, which means I can easily choke. Also, since then, I've developed cancer.

After my lung operation, I spent a year in convalescence at Val David. When I felt well again, I was asked to take on a house for novices. Later, I was also asked to help out with the older sisters who were sick and dying. Without realizing it, I had taken on too much and was pushing myself too hard. I was getting more and more worn out, more and more tired, but was paying no attention to myself. I acted as if nothing was wrong with me. Then I got three colds in a row. In my condition, that was quite dangerous. I had to return to Val David for four more years of convalescence. During that time, I also helped out where I could. It was impossible to stop being active. My style was not to just sit around and calmly relax.

My other problem began around the time of the tuberculosis. I started to develop arthritis of the spine, at the base of the neck. Now the vertebrae in my neck have fused together, and the nerves have no room. They're squeezed. That can be very painful. The pain starts in the neck and rises to the top of the head, to the left. For the past five years, every single night I have woken up in the middle of the night in pain. At times I can make it to four in the morning without waking up. I begin by sleeping in bed, and after three or four hours I wake up, take painkillers, and move to the chair to continue my sleep. I can take only one painkiller every four hours, which means my ability to live through the night is truly put to the test. Before going to sleep, I sign a blank check to God. I say, "The night is yours, You know what's best." No two nights are the same. But by the afternoon, the pain goes away. This is my load to carry, a form of exercise to strengthen my shoulders. Others have a different load.

More and more, the pain brings to mind the question of love. I have often spoken about the importance of love. I thought I knew all its varieties but now find myself probing, analyzing its different facets. One has to love others. One has to allow oneself to be loved. And one must learn to receive God's love, which is explosive, dynamic, overflowing. We are rarely willing or ready to admit such love. These days, I'm learning that each time I say yes to the will of God, my capacity to accept this love grows.

If I don't waste my time worrying about tomorrow and fully live in the present, then I allow myself to be loved. Tomorrow is none of my business. Tomorrow doesn't concern me. It will be a surprise. Everything is a surprise. I have no expectations. I'm not waiting for anything. I try to be in the present moment, and when I find myself in the past or in the future, I bring myself back. This is constant work because my imagination time-travels. I must catch it and bring it back home. God is only in the present, the here and now. All I need to do is remember God, and He will bring me back to the moment. This constant attunement to the Divine is my preparation for death.

Personally, I don't think I would ever be ready to die because I alone cannot prepare for death. God is helping me in this work day to day. When he finds I'm ready, He will come for me. In the meantime, I don't think about death. I think about life.

When I do think of death, I'm afraid because I'm afraid of physical suffering. Suffering is not a creation of God, though He has chosen it as a vehicle to enter deeper into His love. Suffering strengthens faith and trust. When I have a bad headache and have done everything possible to alleviate it without success, I look at Jesus with his crown of thorns and say, "You never had any painkillers."

I find all sorts of little tricks to forget the pain. One night I went to Nazareth. Another night I went to Egypt. Time passed quickly. I don't completely forget the pain, but at least I try to rise above it. I can forget myself a little, and that allows me to live. Of course, I'm discovering that I can only really live when I can love myself. And that's tricky when pain enters the picture. While working with the sick and dying sisters, I was faced with countless examples of how pain can turn one against oneself. Pain can elicit anger, which over-shadows love.

If we love God without loving ourselves, we can never love anyone. True love does not discriminate. In the same way, when I love only myself, I'm only half alive. If my only concern is my little person, my world is small. To be fully alive, in life, the ideal is to love God and His creation equally, which includes other people as well as oneself. That is a deceptively simple notion. It has virtually taken me my whole life to be able to put that into practice. For me the love of God came naturally. The love of others was also there, though that needed considerable expansion. To fully understand the love of self has taken me almost my whole life.

It hasn't been very long since I've understood that God loves me as I am. Before, I wasn't certain that I would appear before God as I should, as would be expected. And the feeling that God accepts and loves me exactly as I am is still new. I sometimes fall back into fear and think, "I'm not worthy enough to appear before Him." But now that I'm sure God is there for people who are not leading an exemplary life, for the poor, for the sick, for the sinners, I feel better. I feel perfectly comfortable in the company of the poor, the sick, and the sinners. I'm happy to be a sinner. God doesn't ask for perfection. We expect ourselves to be perfect because of our education and society.

When we arrive before God, the only question He will ask us is if we have loved. To love well is the most important achievement we can accomplish here on earth. And to cultivate the seed of love takes time. It takes time till the roots grow deep enough to reach the heart. Theoretically, with my head, I always knew love was the most important aspect of life. That knowledge finally reached my heart through constant readings of the Bible, where the word of God is like love letters to humanity.

I once heard a priest say that from the head to the heart is as far as from New York to Tokyo. I thought that because I knew a lot of things, I also lived them. It has taken me all these years to finally learn that to know is not enough. Only recently has my knowledge shifted from my head to my heart. Was it necessary for me to become almost immobile before this could happen?

Now I see that one of the most important feats in life is to accept oneself, to accept one's limits, one's needs, one's faults. For God, these are not important. Faults and limitations do not bother him. God is not a part of our time system. He does not see things in time. He is in eternity. He's not in a hurry. He doesn't need to rush you. He works patiently, constantly, within every human being.

Since I know that God loves me as I am, I love myself as I am. Before, I loved myself less because I felt I had to be otherwise. I felt I had to be better before God could love me. Now, when I make a mistake, I think, I've forgotten to ask for His help. But I don't break my head over it, I don't worry about it. I acknowledge the error and accept that I have hit my limit. I no longer blame myself for it.

Before entering the order, I idealized nuns. To me, they seemed perfect. When I was going to school for my teaching diploma, I looked at the nuns, and they always seemed so happy and fulfilled. There was never any friction between them. I thought, When I enter the order I'll also be perfect.

But soon after becoming a novice, I realized I had entered the order with my faults. Later, it occurred to me that since I had faults, surely I'm not the only one. Of course God has never said that in order to be a nun you must not have any faults, you must be perfect. One day I woke up to the discovery that nuns were simply ordinary people. Sisters are also human beings. It was an astonishing revelation.

It wasn't until the age of twenty-three, when I entered the order, that I began to find faults in others as well as in myself. At times, I saw faults in others, whereas I ignored those same faults in myself. Once I had a good laugh at my own expense. A group of us were playing cards, and one of the sisters was quite distracted. The sister beside her was getting more and more impatient. I thought to myself, "She should be more tolerant."

Three minutes later, it was I who was getting impatient. I saw it right away. I said, Angela, it's your turn. Stop judging others. Often I was very severe and judgemental when I saw someone make a mistake. I never verbalized my judgements, except on the rare occasion when I felt the other person could benefit from them, but I certainly felt them internally.

I think this judgemental side grew out of my idealism. And my idealism developed at an early age. I was the youngest of twelve children and was always called the last little one. I was very much loved and very much spoiled. The last little one looked at the bigger ones and found them wonderful. I saw only their good qualities. As I grew up, I presumed everyone to be like them. Perfect.

Living in the community has taught me that we are all human beings who have not yet matured. And it is important to allow others to be where they are, to accept them as they are. If necessary, to wait for them patiently. There is no rush for them to be anywhere else.

I have become much more tolerant since I've looked at my own shortcomings and discovered my limits. And I'm happy to know that I have limits. Each time I discover a new one, which is almost every day, I say to God, "Thank you."

I think one of the reasons it has taken me so long to realize that God loves me exactly the way I am is due to a little error, perhaps on the part of my parents, who thought one must be perfect to stand before God. One must be pure. For instance, before I went to communion, I absolutely had to go to confession first. Everything had to be forgiven. As a result of this religious teaching, I think our ancestors, my parents and grandparents, had more anxiety than necessary about approaching God.

My father was more confident before God. He was not a rich man, but we always had everything we needed. The farm where we lived had belonged to my paternal grandparents. My father worked the land with my brothers' help. He never ordered my eight brothers to do anything. He suggested a possible course of action, and everyone was happy to do it. Our house was open to everyone. Our family was like everyone's family. My father was a very considerate man who had no enemies in a community where everyone knew everyone. He was a man who loved and lived in peace. Everyone liked him. At the age of sixty-six, on Christmas Day, he came to visit me when I was still a novice. On the tenth of January, 1941, he died. He had been sick for only ten days. His last words were, "I offer my life to peace in the community and the world." I wasn't there, but James, my older brother, who was by then a priest, was there.

Unlike my father, my mother was quite anxious about being good enough or pure enough to stand before God. Today we would say she was a perfectionist. Back then, the constant effort to purify one-self was considered a virtue. Of course, this incessant self-purification meant you had to keep looking for faults within yourself.

Traditionally, it was recommended that you go to confession once a month. And we went. When I was living with my parents, I confessed little peccadilloes, trifles. Today I understand that the sacrament of forgiveness comes from God's love and grace. I don't think I fully understood it then, at such a young age. At that time, it felt more like housecleaning, like sweeping the floor of dirt.

So I grew up never being certain if God loved me the way I was, and it wasn't until recently that I realized this. Yes, I never quite felt that I was good enough to stand before God. But gradually I realized, not so long ago, that it was God who was the first to love me, and this love in no way depended upon my being perfect. This love depended totally on Divine generosity and acceptance. And it was totally free. It had no price tag.

About ten years ago, I began to understand that there was something about my relationship to God that still needed to be explored. Somehow I felt there was still something I needed to learn. As I meditated and prayed, I began to understand that God chose me as I was and as I am. Through prayer, meditation, and time in retreats, I discovered that God loved me no matter how I was. And I certainly feel I have been chosen by Him to serve.

Why was my older sister, who I found much more perfect than I was, not chosen? She was my godmother as well as my teacher. When I was eight or nine I was a student at the school where she taught. She was a wonderful teacher, and I loved school. Watching her teach with such care and love gave me a desire to do the same. When we went home for the weekends, I played school with my young cousins. I taught them everything I had learned. During the week, I lived with my sister at school and was alone with her every night. Even though she was ten years older, she treated me as her best friend. We were very close. I adored her.

Her death was the great trial of my life. It certainly tested my faith. She died at the age of thirty, fifteen days after the death of her husband. The day after he died, she went into hospital, and two weeks later, it was her turn to die. She left six children behind, from age eleven months to eight years.

James was with her in the hospital. He asked her, "If you had a choice between life and death, what would you choose?"

She said, "I would choose death for myself but life for my children." And she died.

Years later, people still came to me and said, "Your sister was the best teacher we ever had."

It was largely due to my sister's influence, watching how she treated her students, that I felt called upon to help those who seemed less happy. I liked to make a basically pessimistic person see the positive side of life. The sisters I lived with forty years ago still remember me, sisters who changed because I was able to help them see the beauty in life. It was probably because of my desire to help that I was given more and more responsibility.

Of course, it was also my sister who had awakened my passion for teaching. After I got my teacher's certificate in 1936, I taught primary school in a nearby town. I had students from grade one to grade seven, all in the same class. It wasn't easy teaching seven grades at once. At times I got the older students to help the younger ones. The first year I had thirteen students, and with each passing year I had more and more.

My love of teaching is what attracted me to a teaching community of nuns. James had told me about the order of St. Anne. As my sister had helped to awaken my love of teaching, James was instrumental in nourishing my spiritual side. He is seventeen years older than me, and when I was small he often took care of me and played with me. Since he went to Vermont to become a priest, he has written me a letter every month. He comes and spends his holidays with me. When I mention a problem I have, he replies with one sentence, and I immediately have my answer. He says, "Everything comes from God, even that which doesn't seem to make sense. Just tell yourself, God sees something in that." He has been my spiritual counsellor and still is to this day, at the age of ninety-five.

I taught school for four years before entering the order. Joining the community was a big sacrifice because I was very attached to my family. I probably could have continued to be a teacher in ordinary life, but God had given me a taste of something much more grand. I remember one Sunday when I was twelve. Some of the family went off to church. The rest stayed home, since the carriage wasn't big enough for all of us to go. When Mass was due to start, we all kneeled down to pray. My mother had given me a prayer book which contained a chapter called, "Make Me a Saint, My Lord." It was a two-page prayer asking God to make you a saint. I spent one hour just on those two pages. Basically all the prayer said was, "Lord, make me a saint. If I'm a saint I could give more glory to eternity. If I'm a saint I would teach others to love You. If I'm a saint . . ."

I asked to be a saint. I didn't know what it really meant, but this prayer touched me very deeply. Later I said to myself, That was the beginning of my calling. God already had His eyes on me.

When I was in the convent at around age sixteen, we went to Mass every morning. Two mornings in a row, I experienced an overwhelming feeling of love and such joy that I cried and cried, till I finally said, "Enough, God, I'm going to burst and die from joy."

Later, I thought to myself, I must have been a tough nut to crack to have had to be given such a deep experience. Maybe without that experience I wouldn't have understood. I still remember so clearly. I felt such all-pervasive and overwhelming joy. I thought everyone felt this way.

One Sunday afternoon, when I had already joined the community of St. Anne, we went to vespers. While reading a prayer, I lost all sense of place and time. I was everywhere and nowhere. It was a half-hour of pure happiness. I thought we were all so blessed and fortunate. Coming back from vespers, I heard a girl say, "Damn vespers!"

I said to myself, I guess she didn't have the same experience I did. Why did I have that special feeling?

I thought of becoming a nun at a fairly young age. I saw my parents work, my brothers and sisters work. I saw them choose their partners. I went to their weddings. And I remember thinking, I can't see myself married. I felt God had called me to serve Him. That was quite a surprise because I didn't find myself worthy of Him. I think God called me because He simply loved me. He loved me, as He loves everyone. But unlike most I actually experienced that love and wanted to respond. From the first moment I felt God's love, I was willing to follow Him. I didn't know what plans He had for me, nor did I ask. I discovered them day to day. Now I can look back at my life and see everything He has done. I know it is God who has made my life.

I did have a boyfriend for six months before entering the order, but my feelings for God were much stronger than my feelings for him. Finally I told him I was going to become a nun. That ended the relationship. But I was very glad to have known him, otherwise I might have always had a doubt. Now I can honestly say I have never regretted entering the order. I have never missed not having children — I had a lot of children as a teacher, other people's children. I have never thought that being a nun was not enough. I have always felt this was my place.

When I first arrived at St. Anne's as a young teacher, there were forty-five sisters. I felt uncomfortable with forty-four of them. There was one with whom I felt more at ease because we had gone to the same school. I looked upon the others as being very wise, and I felt like the ignorant little girl. Also, I was very shy. I had come from a family where I considered the others to be very important. I was the last little one. I had nothing to offer and nothing important to say. The others always had interesting experiences to relate, and I was more than glad to listen. To me they were all intelligent, wise, and witty.

I wrote to my brother and asked, "How can I overcome my shyness?"

He answered, "First of all, you are no more stupid than the next person. Second, when you make a mistake, don't dwell on it for three days. Turn the page and know you'll do better next time. God has forgotten it, so should you. Third, as long as the other person doesn't tell you you're boring, there's no reason for you to think so. If you have nothing to say, ask questions and be interested in the reply. Remember, Jesus was humble." It took me four months to test his suggestions and to overcome my shyness. Four months later, I spoke to everyone.

When I first entered the order, I taught different grades. Later, I was asked to teach the girls who were applying to join the order. Then I taught the novices for a few years. After that I was asked to be the headmistress for the applicants, where I welcomed the girls. I remember that period with great fondness.

The applicants came dressed in a variety of colours. Upon entering the order, they put on the black habit with the headdress. Before they put on the habit, I learned all of their names. Two days after they arrived, I could call each of them by name. They were surprised and very pleased.

The girls who applied to be nuns were supple, eager to learn and be better. They were still idealistic. It was very satisfying to see them develop. Each girl was unique, an individual. Early on, I realized I couldn't like all of them equally. I prayed that I would never develop a dislike toward any of them. I felt it would be unfair to only judge the girls by external appearances or to dislike one because of a personality difference. When one girl seemed less interesting than the others, she would be the first to whom I gave my attention. And I found wonderful qualities in all of them. All of them had a certain internal beauty. Still today I remember their names. All the details about them are faithfully recorded in my mind. I can't forget any of them.

When I was forty-five, after having worked for eight years with the applicants, I was asked to be a Mother Superior. That was a real test for me. I had a great respect for the Mother Superior of a convent. I always put her on a pedestal, kept her at a respectful distance. And that wasn't my style at all. I looked at the older Mother Superiors and thought, I will never be able to do this. Becoming a Mother Superior seemed so foreign to me. But in those days you weren't asked if you wanted a particular post. You were simply told, This is what you have to do. I didn't have a choice.

I was told to go to a special retreat for Mother Superiors. And I was very nervous. Finally I said to myself, Since the authorities believe I can do it, I will at least try. But I didn't have much confidence.

To my surprise I found that the very qualities I considered important as a teacher helped me to become a good Mother Superior. I deemed each person important. I made an effort to treat everyone equally and felt each one deserved respect.

I was responsible for the community as a Mother Superior for twenty years. Just because we have all chosen to become nuns doesn't mean we love God in the same way. The faces of love are infinite. There are different ways, different approaches to God. At first, I was very surprised to discover not all the sisters loved God the way I did. Not all the sisters tried to enter the mystery of God and life as I did. Therefore, I didn't find many people on the same spiritual level as myself, people with whom I could share and explore my spiritual search. That was a disappointment.

Still, since I have entered the community I have always had a few good friends. These friendships, which have been basically spiritual in nature, have very much enriched my life. Of course, there was also a personal part to the friendship where we shared our difficulties and tried to help each other find answers. But it always started because we loved God in a similar way. We both had a desire to be united with God. I think this is why the friendships were as strong as they were. God is not absent from friendships. He can be giving you help through your friend. The Bible says Jesus also had friends. He even had preferences. Among his twelve disciples, John was his favourite.

My friendship with Louise started when she told me she had become so devoted to teaching that it had overtaken her life. There was no room for God.

"I have no energy to give to God during prayer time," she said. "Everything I have goes to teaching. My desire to teach well has become all-pervasive."

She had become too preoccupied with the human plane, the physical level. She came to me as the Mother Superior to ask for guidance on how to re-establish her contact with God. I gave her some suggestions. She tried them out and regularly came back to ask me more questions. She continued to work on herself, to clear an inner space where she could reconnect to God. She kept coming back to talk to me. She made tremendous progress on the spiritual path. After four years we became very close. We had some wonderful spiritual discussions where we searched for answers together.

Since I've been in the infirmary, I've had more spiritual discussions than ever before. Now I often talk about God with people who come to visit. Also, the sisters know this is the topic that most interests me at this stage of my life, and they come to my room specifically to talk about spiritual matters. I'm surprised at how many people want and seem to need to talk about the Divine. A sister who is now blind and eighty-two years old regularly pays me a visit. Our discussions are always spiritual in nature. I also enjoy hearing about other people's experiences. They help me in my own search. Perhaps now, more than ever, I have a thirst to enter into the Divine Mystery.

Day to day, I learn how to love God better and how to better understand and love others. Every human being is an individual. Each heart is beautiful, rich and contains a treasure. And I have not yet mined all the hearts, have not yet discovered the treasures within each. Before, as Mother Superior, I spent considerable time listening to people. Now I also listen, but with a difference. I no longer listen to the words. I listen to the spirit and the heart.

Last week the nurse said to me, "You don't go out of your room very often. You seem to have cut yourself off."

I said, "If you could only know. I have never felt more at one with the whole world since I've come here." Visitors bring me news. They talk about their work, and they ask me to pray for them. Now my work is to help people with my prayers.

Being sick and bedridden is like day and night compared to the daily life of a community. A working community is very much alive, everyone has a job to do. Each one comes back at night to discuss the day's activities over supper. If someone has a problem, everyone tries to help her with both advice and prayer. Here, in the infirmary, there is a tendency to be preoccupied with one's own health. People no longer have the energy to think of others. Yet for me, I find this is a wonderful opportunity for inner expansion, for the cultivation of that inner silence where God speaks. Also, it is in my immobile state that I'm learning to serve others in a different way.

At the beginning of each year every sister of St. Anne receives a letter stating her task for the year. This year my task is to minister prayers. In other words, I pray to help others get closer to God. When I was at Val David in convalescence, my task was community service, whatever service I could offer as a receptionist, doing a little housework, sewing.

Right now, prayer is the most important part of my life, and I thank God for whatever happens. At the same time, I ask God to increase my faith. Of course, you have to want to have faith, and you have to make the effort. You have to desire it. Above all, you must ask for it. Ask and it will be given. If I want more light, more intimacy with God, a greater desire for the Divine, I must ask. These are all gifts He wants me to have. But I must make the request.

Faith must be cultivated, nourished, and expanded through acts of love and forgiveness. I have cultivated my faith through trials. At the time I didn't realize it but later I said, "That was a call from God to encourage me to take another step toward faith."

God is always speaking to us through the people and events around us. All we need to do is pay attention and listen. As well, He speaks to us from within. When I extinguish the outside noises, the useless preoccupations, and create an internal silence, I feel Him. He speaks in that inner silence. He does not speak in the noise. If we don't hear Him, it is because the volume of our inner noise is too high. Millions of worries clamour for our attention. One has to live with one's feet on the ground, but some take the ground too seriously. Pascal, a very wise man, wrote, "Life is a light between two eternities."

We live a temporal life and often believe this is all there is. We revel in the pleasures this temporal life has to offer, including the bounty of the earth, but this is not real joy. Real joy comes from accepting God's love and returning that love. Nothing other than that could possibly satisfy us. No other joy can fulfill us.

There is a sister who is around sixty years old, and for the past forty years she's had multiple sclerosis. She can do nothing for herself. She can't even brush away a fly. Yet she is always smiling, always happy. She never complains because she has said yes. She has accepted whatever comes. When we say yes to death, we say yes to life and to God's will. The Divine plan is not death but eternal life. Death is the ultimate communion with God. A passage to eternity. We are meant to live eternally. We are not meant to die.

Our first ancestors passed from temporal life to eternal life without death. Satan introduced death, the break between temporal and eternal life. He has made us forget our origins, and talking of eternal life has become a taboo. But I would hope we could live for God before we die for God. Beyond life is an extraordinary beauty we cannot possibly comprehend while still here on earth. That is what will be real life. When we die we will be born into eternity, eternal beauty. Until then we're living a little life, during which we can seek an intimate contact with God to have a taste of eternity.

Contact with God requires surrender. God allows everyone to freely choose Him or refuse Him. Human beings must choose from a state of absolute freedom. If I ask God to help me surrender to Him, He cannot refuse me.

When I was still a novice, James sent me a pamphlet called, *Peace in Surrender*. It was only two pages long, and it has always been with me. I keep it in my prayer book. It says that Jesus alone is our eternal peace, our divine rest. Don't be moved, impressed, or guided by anyone else but Jesus. This is something I have read every day from the time I received it. It has helped me understand that peace in surrender is the height of love. I have tried to practice it. And still try to practice it. I feel that even today I have not yet fully lived the words of those two pages. When I visited the older sisters who were sick and dying, every time I left their room I said, "I wish us peace in surrender."

Since I have arrived here, in the infirmary, I have said to myself, Angela, you are here to live peace in surrender. It helps me to live each moment. Each instant I try to surrender to what God gives me. If today He wants me to have a headache, it's a sign of His love, it comes from Him, and I say, Thank you, as I say thank you when He gives me joy.

I will continue to learn about abandonment and surrender till my last breath. I will continue to explore the infinite facets of God's love. We tend to think that, because God gives us trials and obstacles, He doesn't love us, but that's not true. He wants us to be happy. God wants us to find Him in the darkness. It is from God that all light comes. I call to God every day, I cry for Him to come to me.

I pray that the Holy Ghost open the doors of my heart till my whole being is flooded with light. Of course, first the desire has to be there. St. Theresa of Avila said, "Ask for the desire from Desire." All you have to do is desire and already it becomes a reality. Of course, you also have to have faith. Everything hinges on faith. Through faith we feel His love. And life is but a journey where we learn about love.

All the love that has existed since the beginning of creation is a spiritual treasure to which each person adds a little. This treasure is accessible to everyone, even to those who do not believe in its existence. In that sense, every human being is saved.

As long as I'm breathing, I will continue to learn to love more and more, and, hopefully, I will be able to contribute to this spiritual treasure. In the present, I try to stay as open as possible to the wishes of God. From day to day, I work at allowing God to prepare me for the end, without my interference. When He says my life is over and this body will die, then the circle of my temporal life will close. Till then, my task is to expand my capacity to give and receive love.

I don't ask what's going to happen or how it's going to happen. I don't need to know. God knows. And I no longer look at death but at a new life that's about to start.

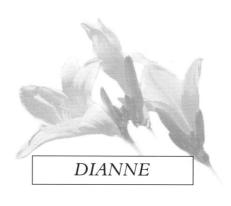

DIANNE

Before giving me her name, the hospital psychologist told me that Dianne was someone special to her, and she had done something she would normally never do. Good friends of hers were looking for a child to adopt. Dianne, thirty-five, was looking for an appropriate couple to adopt her child before her death from AIDS. *The psychologist arranged for Dianne and her friends to meet. The couple adored Dianne and her child, and after they had become well acquainted, they agreed to adopt him after she died. The psychologist was certain Dianne would be willing to talk; she would be interested in putting her life in perspective.*

The psychologist was right. Dianne agreed to see me. I went to her small apartment on the second floor of a duplex in a modest area. She had made the appointment for a time when her son would be in school and we would be free to talk. She was reserved yet open. Slim and attractive, with short blond hair, she was casually dressed in slacks and a T-shirt. I could sense the passion behind her reserve.

For the third interview, I went to her house with biscotti that I had made. Dianne was very sick. The interview would have to be postponed. She asked me if I would drive her to emergency. We sat in the waiting room of the hospital with other sick people. She was nervous, understandably anxious. So was I. She did not voice the obvious. I am

*certain we both thought this could be the end. Two hours later, her
name was called.*

*The next time I saw her, she was on a hospital bed in the corridor.
She was not happy; the hospital was going to hold her. This was
already after one o'clock in the afternoon. I remembered the biscotti
in my purse, and I gave them to her. She gladly took them and said
she would call me as soon as they let her out. I was afraid I would
never hear from her. I didn't want to visit her in the hospital. I didn't
want to interfere with her relatives and her children, and how would
she explain me? I kept in touch with her social worker, who knew
what was happening. Two weeks later, she did call.*

*I usually went to her house at ten o'clock in the morning for our
interview. The fourth time, she invited me to stay for lunch. Her son
had come home to eat. She introduced me and explained who I was
in an adult way, not using baby talk, not overtly coddling.*

*She washed an apple for him, vigorously rubbing all parts of it
with her palms, as I do today after Dianne's example, making sure the
running water had touched every area. She served his food with care
and love, yet efficiently and quickly, and answered questions calmly
and reasonably. I was impressed.*

*During the next interview, when she was telling me she had done
research into what quick and painless pill to take for suicide, I asked
her to name it. She refused to tell me. I did not push, thinking she was
right not to answer such a question.*

Four years ago, my husband was taken to hospital by ambulance. He
had a high fever and was delirious. Ten days later, on Easter Sunday,
my sister-in-law called to say Kevin had died of a heart attack. She
also said he might have had AIDS. That was a jolt. We had been
separated for six months, and I thought the separation might only be
temporary.

I couldn't reach the doctor till the following Tuesday. On the
phone I said, "I hear Kevin might have died of AIDS. How is that
possible?"

He said, "Your son was bisexual so he was easily at risk."

I was stunned. I couldn't say a word.

The doctor thought I was his mother. After a long silence, he asked, "To whom am I speaking?"

"To his wife."

"I'm sorry. We have to talk. Come to my office in three days. By then I'll have the autopsy results."

The autopsy results showed that Kevin had had pneumonia, and there were bacteria specific to AIDS in his lungs. The doctor suggested I go for tests, along with Justin, who was ten months old at the time. There was no way to tell when Kevin got the virus. Maybe while we were together, or maybe even before. Both Justin and I could easily have been infected.

My husband had never given me a clue about his sexual orientation. To have learned it after his death made me furious. Then I began to remember certain events. We had rented two spare rooms to boarders. At one time, we had a tenant in his early twenties, called Richard. Soon after he arrived, Kevin said to me, "Why don't you go camping? It would do you good. I'll stay in Montreal."

When I came back, he said, "I had a really interesting conversation with Richard. He told me he takes coke. But he's really sharp. I like this guy. We talked in his room till well after midnight."

A few months later, Richard left without paying the rent. Then reappeared and wanted to move back in. I was against it. Kevin insisted on taking him back, giving him another chance. At the time, I thought nothing of it.

I didn't rush out to have the test. I wasn't anxious for the results. Finally I decided that if Justin does have the virus, there might still be time to treat him, in which case I should do this as soon as possible. The doctor sent us to the Children's Hospital, where we were both tested. Then there was the three week waiting period for the results.

In the meantime, Kevin was cremated. I didn't go to the funeral. His family didn't want me there. They blamed me for his death because I had left him. I was the bad one. After the cremation, I went to the funeral parlour to pick up his death certificate, which was legally mine. As I sat waiting in the parlour, I looked at the urns on display. When the woman appeared with the death certificate, I asked her into which urn my husband's ashes had been put. She said, "It's not any of those on display. His ashes are in the most simple container we have." I asked to see it.

She brought out a little black plastic box. Like a black, opaque Tupperware box. At that point, my anger toward Kevin dissipated. I thought, He had had such a miserable life, with such an unhappy childhood, and he ended up, at the age of thirty-five, in a cheap plastic box. It was pitiful.

But I certainly had plenty to be angry about. From the time I had left him I had another court case on my hands. Kevin had wanted custody of Justin. This time, I decided, no matter what, Justin was going to stay with me. I didn't want to repeat the same story as with Isabel. I left with my son on a Friday and had an appointment with a lawyer for Monday. I immediately asked for custody. Again I had to spend $10,000 in lawyer's fees, had to go through a barrage of psychological tests, and had to appear before the judge. Exactly what I went through with Peter, my first husband.

The whole process took three agonizing months, during which time Kevin was constantly threatening to take Justin away from me. He kept insisting that I go back to him for Justin's sake. He kept asking, "Do you want your son to have the same life as your daughter?" Guilt is a powerful weapon.

There were only three months between the time I won custody of Justin and when Kevin died. Another tension-filled three months. During that time, I had constant contact with him because he had visiting rights to our son. And he continually criticized me as a mother. He said Justin was regressing in his development because of me. I was always afraid he might run away with him. He never brought him back on time. I was constantly waiting, pacing, biting my nails. To a certain extent, when Kevin died I was relieved.

While we were together, I was perpetually on edge for fear he might fall into the same violent pattern he had experienced at home. I was afraid Kevin might hit Justin because his own father had physically abused his children. Justin was a good baby, a naturally happy child who always smiled. But a few nights I arrived home from work and found him very agitated, breathless. I was routinely checking him for marks on his body.

When the doctor had the test results, he called me in. He said, "I have good news and bad news." Just like that.

I said, "I guess the good news is, my son doesn't have the virus. The bad news is, I have it."

He nodded. He also added that Justin's results were uncertain. The virus could still develop in a baby up to the age of eighteen months. This meant I had six months to bite my nails and make plans. Even though I had a six-year-old daughter, I decided to commit suicide with Justin if it turned out he had developed the virus. I didn't want the two of us to be submitted to slow torture till we died.

By this time my blood count was already very low. I had full blown AIDS. That's one of the reasons I fell into a panic and had a crisis. I saw Kevin die in ten days. I thought I could probably die just as quickly. Who was going to take care of Justin if I died first? Suicide was the only answer. I wasted no time. I did research into how to commit suicide in the fastest and least painful way possible. I didn't want a failed suicide attempt. I found a place in the woods where we could do it, and it would take them weeks to find us. I had every-thing planned. Except the information I required was not easy to obtain. Finally, in desperation, I called a help line. It seemed the safest route, since it was totally anonymous.

By then I was ready to crack. Time was passing, and I had no time to waste. At last I got the information I wanted. But I was crazy with worry. First because I had to wait for Justin to reach eighteen months, and then I still had to wait three weeks for the results. Before I got Justin's results, I called the help line several more times. Each time I called, the person on the line asked if I wanted to meet other women with AIDS. To talk to them, see how they felt. Each time I took down the necessary information and did nothing.

When I finally got Justin's results, they turned out to be HIV negative. I cried with relief. And decided he needed me to stay alive as long as possible. I had to be there for him. I was the only one left to love him. His father was already dead.

At this point, I called the number I had taken down and joined a group of women who also had AIDS. We met once every two weeks in the presence of a psychologist. At first I thought I was joining people who shared the same disease as myself. Slowly I realized I had joined a therapy group. Our discussions moved from talking about the illness to examining our lives before the illness. All the women present had a history. We were not just women with AIDS. We had all experienced considerable emotional pain, and this illness was simply the last straw.

Two women I later befriended had similar childhoods to mine. All three of us had played with the idea of suicide. Death seemed like a solution in face of difficulties. When, numerous times in your life, you seriously want to die, the desire never totally leaves you. And if little things happen to reactivate it, it remains very much alive in the subconscious. Now that I'm facing the reality of death, after having wished for it a few times in my life, I think, No, I didn't mean it. I wasn't serious.

But the flip side of this crazy situation is that AIDS has allowed me to appreciate life as never before.

As a result of therapy I'm finally beginning to understand myself. Understanding has given me the necessary distance to watch my reactions and to consciously change certain behavioural patterns. Before getting the virus, I would never have gone to a psychologist. I was too independent to need anyone's help. Also, I wouldn't have had the time. I was constantly running.

Two years ago, I stopped working. I stopped just before I was due to be promoted to sales representative, with a salary of $55,000, a position I had been working toward for a number of years. I had put in extensive overtime, even while Justin was very young. I got up at five in the morning, rushed to prepare breakfast, rushed to dress him, rushed to get him to daycare. I ran for the bus and arrived at work breathless. Then I had to deal with problems, with major clients like corporations, airlines. I was always rushing. After work, I picked up Justin from daycare. I went shopping. Cooked dinner. I couldn't get to bed before eleven. The next morning, I was up again at five. Always running. Working in sales requires high-powered performance, which means constant stress. And stress is the worst thing for this illness. I was getting more and more tired and ended up consulting the company doctor. He suggested that I stop working, since my immune system was so weak. I left on prolonged sick leave without telling anyone what I had. Now the insurance allows me to live a little above the poverty line. I have just enough money to eat, pay rent, and not much more.

After two years of not working, I'm finally beginning to appreciate my freedom. I've learned to listen to my body and not push it beyond its limits till I fall flat on my face. I take time to live, to breathe. When working, you're thinking about yesterday, tomorrow, upcoming summer holidays. You're constantly thinking about other than the present. In the present, all you feel is stress.

But I loved my work. I adored the challenge of setting up a large telephone system for a company. When the system was in place, it was because I had been the one to oversee all the stages. I had solved all the problems. It was due to me that an established corporation could have a large phone system. It validated my sense of worth. I was indispensable. And I would go to any lengths to get the job done right. I never thought about my own health. I liked what I was doing and didn't listen to my body, which was tired, or to my nerves, which were on edge. This accumulated stress needed an outlet, and it came out as anger at home, anger at the smallest things because I was so tired.

Eight years ago, I even ended up getting pneumonia because I was working too hard. I had to be off work for a month and a half and was penalized. The company doesn't look favourably upon those who are sick. They consider you weak and a less likely candidate for promotion.

At first, when I stopped working, I missed it. I missed the pressure and the tension. It was exciting, a high. But it was an excitement that was totally fuelled by the outside. Since this illness, therapy has taught me to look inside, to examine my feelings and emotions and to take them seriously. I have never done that before in my life. In my family, we talked for hours about the weather, news, politics. Never about feelings, emotions.

As a result, the outside became much more important than the inside, even when I was young. I remember when I was five or six I went into the fields and fell into a puddle. I was covered with mud. I was so afraid my mother would be angry at me for having dirtied my beautiful green dress that by the time I arrived home I had peed in my pants. And, sure enough, she was furious. She punished me by forcing me to stay in my room for four days. I even had to eat my meals there.

As an adult, my house had to be perfect. I bought quality furniture. If the table got scratched, I promptly bought a new one. If the couch had a tear, I replaced it. If the paint on the wall peeled, I immediately had it repainted. I cleaned the windows every week with a special spray. I couldn't tolerate a spot. I wore designer clothes. With every season, I changed my wardrobe. The children had to be dressed perfectly. Isabel's hair had to be just right. Her clothes always had to be clean. Everything around me had to be in order. Perfect. But I still wasn't perfect. And never could be, no matter how hard I tried.

Now that I have AIDS, I will never be perfect, and it's in this state of obvious imperfection that I have learned to finally appreciate myself. Not to blame myself. Before, if my mother didn't love me, it was my fault. If my father didn't love me, it was my fault. If I lost custody of my daughter, it was my fault. I thought everything was my fault. I've tried to be perfect and never could. That's why I was always running, always angry, frustrated. I was never good enough, perfect enough.

Before, even if people loved what I cooked, I always criticized it. Not enough of this or that spice. Overcooked or undercooked. Too much salt or not enough salt. It didn't matter how much other people liked it, I always found fault with it. I now allow myself to make a meal that is not perfect. When people come to visit, I no longer feel everything must be spotless. I'm now capable of paying more attention to the person I'm with than to my surroundings. Sometimes, one needs a crisis to wake up and recognize what's important. Obviously, I needed a very intense crisis.

Having spent the past three years in therapy, I'm now beginning to understand why I acted the way I did. My need for external control was due to a lack of internal control. I was an angry and aggressive perfectionist. I was also an idealist. My boyfriends had to be the ideal boyfriends, and of course I was always disappointed. My friends had to be the ideal friends. If I found one fault, I broke off the friendship. I couldn't allow anyone to have faults. I put people on a pedestal, and they always fell. Then I just left them on the ground.

I was constantly frustrated and angry at my inability to find or attain perfection. My anger came out at home. I threw dishes. I broke whatever I could get my hands on. I frightened even Kevin. I was a terror behind the wheel of a car. If anyone dared to cut me off, I would lower my window and swear at the top of my lungs at the other driver.

At work, I was aggressive in an almost masculine way. I always wanted to know how things worked and why. If a technician said something couldn't be done, I never accepted it. I always asked why. I always asked questions. The only place where I didn't ask questions was in my family. If my mother said something, no matter how irrational, I never challenged her.

When I was young, I tried to make my mother happy. She was an esthetician and had opened her own business. She worked almost twenty-four hours a day. Since she worked so hard and was always tired, I wanted to help her by cleaning the house, washing the floors. I was eight or nine when I began vacuum-cleaning the house. And she was never satisfied. She pointed out that I had forgotten to dust a table or hadn't scrubbed the toilet or hadn't cleaned out the breadbox, or I had forgotten to put out a fresh roll of toilet paper. I got scolded for not having done something instead of being praised for what I did. I was cleaning the house and cooking, and she still wasn't happy.

In spite of her criticism, I thought my mother was wonderful, someone who could do no wrong. I never answered back to her. Instead, I had a few blackouts at school. Each time I came to, the teacher was shaking me and telling me to calm down and then I saw I had destroyed everything around me.

My mother was frustrated, unhappy, and she needed me. She began to confide in me around the time I started to clean the house. She told me about her terrible childhood with her stepmother. She told me how she loved my father and had been disappointed in him, first because he was an alcoholic and second because he was cheating on her. She told me she had found his address book with all these women's names and numbers. She found his diary, in which he had written that his wife wasn't important to him. When she spoke about my father, who had hurt her so much, I thought it was terrible. I wanted him to leave her alone, not to make her so unhappy. On the rare occasion when he was home, he was very impatient, often angry, swore a lot, and criticized everything. I hated him. My parents finally separated when I was eleven.

I was fourteen when Larry entered the picture, and I thought he would replace my father, who had never been there. I had always wanted a father. I thought, Finally I will have one. At last we're going to be a family. We're going to go out together to see movies. I had these idealistic expectations, and then nothing. Larry showed no interest in me. He wasn't like a father and my mother ceased being a mother. Till Larry arrived, I had played the role of psychologist for her, then she no longer needed me. She stopped paying attention to me. I was dispensable, and she threw me away. I didn't even have the comfort of having my sister, who was two years younger than me. My parents had always encouraged the differences between us. They pitted one against the other. As a result, we always fought. And now I felt totally abandoned.

Larry and my mother set up house in the garage, which had been renovated and turned into a bachelor apartment. This separate unit had a bedroom, a den, a bathroom, and a kitchenette. This was where they lived, while we lived in the other part of the house. When he came home from work, he immediately went to his area. When she came home, she also went there. Since she continued to work, she was still always tired. I continued to clean and cook. I cooked for the whole family, but we never ate together. My mother came up to get supper and took it to their apartment. I think one of the reasons we didn't do anything together was because she was jealous of me when Larry moved in. She regularly called from work to ask, "What are you doing? What is Larry doing?"

Once I told him I liked the shirt he happened to be wearing. My mother was immediately upset and said, "Don't compliment him."

Since I had such a difficult time growing up, my attraction to the mystical was like my faith. When I was eight or nine, I found a book my aunt had lent my mother. It was about the history of the world, the pyramids, initiations, angels, God. I was so intrigued I read it twice from cover to cover. Since then, I've been going to libraries and reading anything I could find on spirituality and mysticism. Sometimes I read the Bible, just because I liked it. I've always been attracted to ancient Egypt, the pyramids, the history of the pharaohs. From time to time I saw Egyptian hieroglyphics, and I was mesmerized. I didn't understand it, but I was certain if I looked long enough and hard enough I would be able to decipher its meaning. It seemed so familiar.

I wanted to be an archeologist, but my mother decided that wasn't a very lucrative profession. She said, "Listen, even when you have a degree in archeology you might not be able to find work. You might not make money right away. It might be better if you had a stable job."

And I liked nice things. My mother had always bought me beautiful clothes. I couldn't quite see myself living on the poverty line, the way she described it. She suggested I take a secretarial course and sent me out of town to a convent to learn typing and shorthand. Sending me away also solved the problem of my adolescence. Before, she always said, Dianne, do this, eat that, come home at this time, don't play with that friend. And Dianne always listened and obeyed. When I was sixteen I began to rebel.

At the convent, I ran into trouble with the principal and decided to quit. My mother wasn't pleased. When I arrived home, she said, "You have to find a job."

I went to the phone company, and they hired me. Then my mother said, "Now you have to pay rent and contribute to the house."

I had to buy all my personal things like soap and toothpaste. If I wanted to eat something special, I had to pay for it. When I calculated how much it cost me to live at home, I realized I would be better off in my own apartment.

When I was eighteen, on my birthday, I moved out of the house. I left as soon as I was of age and knew the police could no longer come after me. Also, what finally pushed me into action was that I almost strangled my mother. I had forgotten to buy laundry detergent and went down to the basement to take some of hers to do my laundry. Usually we had two boxes of detergent, one with my name on it and one with her name on it. As I was pouring the detergent into a cup, a voice from behind me hissed, "What are you doing?"

I hadn't even heard her approach. I thought I was alone, safe. She started yelling at me. I had a blackout and when I came to, my hands were around her throat. I was shaking her. I immediately let go. She ran away, yelling, "My daughter has gone crazy."

After that I said to myself, "I have to get out of here before I really go crazy."

∞

I saw how my mother had suffered when she found out my father had affairs, and I refused to suffer because of a man. I never wanted to be a wife who waited at home for her husband. Also, I think because my father was never there as I got older, I needed to seduce men. I had to win them. I loved playing the seductress. I always looked my best, always well dressed, perfectly made up, glittering and alluring. Full of wit. Quick on the comebacks. To seduce a man proved I was attractive, I had a certain power over him. I felt very insulted when a man thought he had seduced me. I wanted to be the one doing the seduction. But seducing only one man wasn't enough. I always needed a new one to tell me I was beautiful, sexy, desirable, fun.

First I needed to seduce them, then I had to be certain they loved me. If a man stopped being attentive after a certain time, I found someone else. "How dare you not pay attention to me?"

And I punished him by moving on.

I never gave myself fully to a man. I refused to be at the mercy of love. I was always ready to leave. I didn't want to feel demolished because a man no longer loved me. And I wasn't going to wait around till he stopped loving me. I left before. I needed a love that was passionate, always new. I met someone, it was fun for a while, when it got boring I moved on.

I've always had a man in my life, but only for physical needs and amusement. My affairs usually lasted about two years. Two years of romance, and then I found someone else. I stayed with Peter for four years, but after two years the romance was gone, and I went looking for someone else. I needed the newness, the excitement. Peter never knew. I had a double life. I was able to make a clear distinction between my two lives without any feelings of guilt. At home, I was the wife. Outside, I was the mistress. On one side, my need for stability was fulfilled, and on the other, my need for adventure was fulfilled.

Work provided numerous opportunities for seduction. There were always parties to introduce a new product. There was constantly some new event to celebrate. Sometimes we spent a couple of days in the country to discuss a sales strategy. That was an ideal time to start something.

All the men I chose were either married or had girlfriends. I didn't want them free. I didn't want someone to fall in love with me and want me forever. That's what happened with Peter. When I met him he had no one in his life and he insisted I stay with him. Exactly what I didn't want. I wanted to decide when I would leave a man. I wanted to be in charge.

Peter was a workaholic, and I found myself in exactly the same situation as when I was small. Alone. This time, alone with my daughter. The father who is never there, working all the time. He left early in the morning. He came back late at night. He returned to work after supper. Exactly like my father. And I was very unhappy because I wanted my daughter to have a father. I didn't want her to grow up as I had done. Materially speaking, I had everything I could want. We had a new house, the latest car. I had designer clothes, a good salary. Between the two of us, we brought in over $80,000 a year. And I wasn't happy. Also, I felt I could easily get aggressive, and I was scared. I was often at the point of totally losing my temper. And I didn't want my daughter to see what it was like for a mother and father to fight. As I had seen when I was young. I was getting more and more frustrated and more and more depressed. I didn't know how to change the situation. I felt trapped. It was at this point that I met Kevin.

Before I met him, I had heard about him for ten years from a mutual friend. She always spoke of him as someone quite special, someone who had managed to escape a terrible childhood, had gained control of his life, and was very brave and generous. Always in superlative terms. By the time I met Kevin, I was primed to like him. I found him very intelligent, articulate, and good-looking. He had a good sense of humour. And he readily opened up to me. He told me about the violence he had experienced at home. He had been beaten every day till he was eight years old, and then he set fire to the house because he couldn't take it anymore. He had also been sexually molested as a child by a neighbour. His pain fascinated me. I wanted to give him love and affection, which he never had while growing up. I wanted to give him a little light because he had known such darkness. I gave myself to him to try to make up for all the pain he had suffered during his childhood.

But he also appealed to my need for excitement. He was a man of action. Impulsive. Always ready to do things. A real adventurer with a motorcycle. We went for midnight rides in the country. He had a wonderful sense of romanticism. With Peter, I could do whatever I wanted, alone. He showed me his love by giving me things. And there was Kevin, who was charming, seductive, sexy. I fell for him.

Kevin paid attention to me in a way no one had done before. He asked me how I felt, what I thought. He asked for my opinion. And he listened. No one had ever been interested in my opinion before. And when he took me in his arms and told me he loved me, his words went right to my bones. I truly felt in my body that he loved me. I had never felt that with anyone else.

I decided to leave Peter and think about what I really wanted. I left my daughter with her father and found an apartment. I didn't want to take Isabel with me, away from her father, her babysitter, her toys, her room. I wasn't even sure if the separation would be for good. I thought I might go back. So I didn't want to drag her into uncertainty.

Also, since I never really had a father, it was important for me that Isabel have her father. I so much wanted my daughter to be close to her father that, as soon as she was born and the doctor gave her to me, I immediately passed her on to Peter. I felt that I wasn't really a good enough mother. I felt she deserved something better than me. I was impatient, often angry. I thought Isabel would be much better off with Peter, who I felt was more patient and kind.

When I left the house, I said to myself, "He'll have to take care of her. He won't be able to work such ridiculously long hours. He'll have to devote more time to her." Instead, once I left, he found someone else to take care of her.

When it was clear that I wouldn't go back to Peter, I told him I thought it would be better for Isabel to stay with me. He consulted a lawyer and demanded custody. I also consulted a lawyer. He said he wanted her to stay with him till the court decided her future, and he asked me to pay child support.

Kevin and I moved in together. Before we were due to get married, I realized he was an alcoholic. I told him I refused to marry an alcoholic. He didn't want me to leave and promised to stop drinking before the marriage. And he did. Before, whenever I told a man that I was leaving, he never tried to talk me into staying. All those who claimed to love me always respected my decision to leave. They never argued with me, not even Peter. I think I would have liked them to say, "Listen, I love you, maybe we can work things out." Kevin did that. He stopped drinking for me, cold, without any therapy. And I knew it was hard for him.

The custody case took a year. At the onset, we had told the judge we were going to be married, and Isabel would have a stable home. A few months after we were married the judge asked to speak to Kevin. We went into his chambers, where he opened a file before him and said to Kevin, "This file contains psychiatric reports on you." Kevin had told me he had been in prison for a burglary attempt. In prison, he had had to see various psychiatrists and was given numerous tests. And his criminal record had not yet been erased. In the judge's chambers, it comes out that he had been in prison for an actual burglary, during which he had assaulted a man so badly he had maimed him for life. The judge said, "These reports categorize you as a man who is extremely violent." When I heard this, I immediately knew I would lose the case. No judge will place a four-year-old child in a home where the man has been labelled extremely violent.

Peter got custody of Isabel. The judge said it had nothing to do with me as a mother, it was due to Kevin. I was furious. I told the judge that if he gave Isabel to the father, it wasn't the father who was going to take care of her and raise her because he was never home. It would be the grandmother and babysitters. That's exactly what happened. Soon after I lost custody, I actually thought about having Peter killed.

Though, in retrospect, I must admit I believe it was better for her to have ended up with her father, where she was allowed to be a little girl. I was with Isabel till she was three and a half, and I remember I didn't allow her to be a child. She couldn't make too much noise. She couldn't get dirty. She had to be perfectly clean, perfectly behaved. In therapy, I realized I was doing the same thing with Justin. I can't expect him to be quiet all the time. He's a child. I can't expect him to act like an adult.

One day when Isabel was here for the weekend, she was making a lot of noise, fighting with Justin, talking a lot. She wouldn't listen to me when I told her to be quiet, and I jumped on her, with my fingers around her throat. She was only six at the time. I had never before touched my daughter. I had never hit her. This time, I pushed her against the wall and put my hands around her throat. And something happened to me. I saw myself from a distance and didn't want Isabel to grow up to be like me. Nor did I want to leave an image of a mother who was aggressive, tense, always angry. Soon after that, I was diagnosed with AIDS.

When I entered the women's group, one of the first fears I verbalized concerned my potential violence toward my son. I said to the psychologist, "There is so much violence and anger in me that I'm afraid one day I might do something to him without meaning to."

I felt as if I had been stretched to the limit. Anything more and I would break. There was no more give. I was afraid of losing control. I told him I couldn't take noise. Justin always had to be quiet, and at the time he was not even two. Sometimes I saw myself hitting him and saw him go flying through the air. I never did it, but I saw myself doing it and at times wanted to do it. My head was filled with scenes of violence. But I love my children. I told him what had happened with Isabel and gradually began to talk about my anger.

Soon after that, I started a game with Isabel. At the end of the weekend, I asked her to tell me what she liked most about her visit with me and what she liked the least. When she told me what she liked, I repeated it. And when she told me what she didn't like, I tried not to do it. One day she said, "It really scares me when you're driving and yell at other drivers."

I was surprised. When people honked at me for no reason, I would get out of the car and swear. And I did this even when the children were with me. I asked why that scared her. She said, "I'm afraid one day you'll yell at someone who will hit you."

Ever since then, I'm careful. Now I'm even calm while driving. People can honk at me, they can cut me off, and it's fine. I no longer get angry, all because Isabel told me it scared her and she explained why.

I began paying attention to when my anger erupted. I found myself yelling at Justin if he spilled something on the floor. I would yell at the top of my lungs. I'd become hysterical if a glass was knocked over during a meal. Hysteria was my immediate reaction. I didn't understand it. It's not such a terrible thing if a glass of water or juice or milk is spilled during supper. For me, it was a crisis. Now, I'm no longer so tense. I no longer get angry when there's water on the bathroom floor after he takes a bath. The more perfect I had wanted to be as a mother, the less perfect I became. Now that I'm no longer trying to be perfect, I find I'm a much better mother.

In therapy, I realized I might not be a perfect mother but I'm a mother who is capable of deeply loving her children. Acknowledging that I was capable of such deep love was like a gift to myself. That realization now allows me to take my children in my arms and give of myself emotionally to them. To make them feel my love. The way I felt when Kevin told me he loved me. I felt the truth of his words in my body.

Before Kevin and I got married, it was wonderful. After we got married, it was hell. I was under slow torture from the moment we exchanged vows. He started drinking again. He always got into arguments with friends. He had to be right, no matter what the subject. This wasn't someone who simply said he didn't agree with you. If necessary, he attacked you personally to prove his point. He became verbally violent with me. He would get angry and insulting, and then he would be very affectionate and kind. Then he told me he had physically abused other women. He had broken one girlfriend's finger. I think he thought it was safe to tell me all this once we were married. He thought I couldn't run away. Plus I was already pregnant. Before Justin was born, I was so upset I tried to commit suicide by cutting my wrist. I had just lost my daughter, and I realized I had made a mistake in marrying Kevin. He was not the man I thought he was.

I began to be afraid. Because I was afraid, I became defensive as well as aggressive. Kevin brought out all my aggressivity. I broke dishes. I threw chairs across the room. I even broke a door. This aggressivity scared me because I didn't know how far I was capable of going. Then one night I was so angry with Kevin I actually took a kitchen knife and ran at him. I wanted to kill him. He immediately said to me, in a hauntingly calm voice, "I knew you were going to do that to me one of these days."

That stopped me. It was as if he had wanted to die. That was frightening and incredibly draining emotionally. But I did stay with him for two years before I finally left. I might have been anxious when I was with him, but I was certainly not bored.

The relationship between Kevin and me was very passionate sexually, and passionate in anger as well. I never knew when I woke up in the morning if he would be in a good or bad mood. The pattern of my life. I've always been on this edge of not knowing where I stood. Are my parents going to have a fight today, or is it going to be relatively calm? Are they going to separate, or aren't they going to separate? The air was electric. There was that edge of anticipation, never knowing what will happen. As a result, I think I was attracted to a life filled with tension. I had lived with it when I was young. There was no security, but at the same time it was familiar, even seductive. I found myself in the same dynamic with Kevin. But when I was young, I was the spectator of the drama, even though the drama affected me. With Kevin, I became one of the characters.

Kevin had problems finding a job, and when he did, he couldn't hold onto it. I was the breadwinner in the family. I didn't feel terrific about that. It was Kevin's idea to rent out two rooms to boarders because we needed the money. We had a large place, so the boarders didn't interfere with our lives. Plus he already had experience in renting rooms. Both Kevin and I chose the boarders, who were always men. And he collected the rents. But when I was pregnant, we didn't even have boarders. We were living solely on my earnings.

Kevin regularly asked me for money to go shopping. I gave him fifty dollars, and he came back with no change. He asked for fifty dollars to put gas in the car when I knew it didn't cost that much to fill it up. He said, "I also need to buy something."

I didn't know where all this money was going. Then he got a job working for a pharmacy and stole $300. Of course, he was fired. When he came home, he told me right out what had happened. I asked him why he had to steal the money. He said he needed it to buy coke. Just like that. And there I was pregnant. That was the first time I heard he took coke. I had never had any experience with drug addicts. I didn't know what to do. But now I understood where all the money was going. From then on, I did all the shopping and filled up the car myself. At one point, I asked him to see someone to deal with his violent behaviour. Soon after Justin's birth, he went into therapy for eight months and then stopped because we didn't have enough money. A month later, he tried to choke me.

Before I gave birth to Justin, Kevin was totally there for me. He was remarkable. He massaged my feet, my neck. When I was pregnant with Isabel, Peter didn't know what to do. He was nervous. Kevin took charge. When I was giving birth, he held my hand and kept saying, "Look at me. Look straight into my eyes. Use my strength." And I felt his strength. I felt his love. We maintained eye contact throughout the birth. Justin's birth was like an act of love. I'll never forget his eyes when Justin was born. He just kept gazing at me, eyes moist, filled with wonder.

Justin was like a second gift. I was really pleased he was a boy. I thought, It'll be different with a boy than with a girl. I don't love

Justin more than my daughter. I love him in a different way. I gave him the love I couldn't give to Isabel. I loved to touch him when he was a baby, and I never did that with Isabel. Right from the start, I gave myself to him emotionally. With Isabel, she always had to be well dressed, clean. I was proud of her. But I didn't open to her emotionally.

Soon after Justin was born, Kevin began to lose weight. He was tired all the time. His veins stood out. The colour of his skin had changed. He became very red, his skin was very dry. At the time, I thought the change in his skin colour and the dryness might have been due to bad diet. I knew he wasn't eating well.

One day he asked me for my bank card. I refused to give it to him. Financially, the situation was terrible. I told him I needed the money that was in the account to buy Justin some clothes. He insisted I give him the card. I said, "No!" He became furious and grabbed my throat. He almost choked me. At the time, Justin was six months old, and I didn't want to have violence around him. Nor did I want him to grow up to be like his father, an alcoholic, taking coke, and incapable of shaking himself free of his past. I thought, That's it, never again. I don't want to be part of this violence. Six months after I married him, I left. And three months after I left, he died.

After Kevin died, I didn't have another man for three years. I felt I was now a carrier of death. Before, I always needed to seduce a man to feel desirable. With the virus, I knew I was definitely not desirable. In time, with the help of therapy, I discovered I had to be desirable to myself. I had to learn to accept myself with all my imperfections. And I now see that perfection isn't necessary. Nor is it possible.

All our lives, we're busy suppressing our emotions, and we lose sight of who we are. As a baby, we're given a pacifier to stop us from crying. When depressed, we're told things will get better. We're never encouraged to face the reality of our feelings. As a result, we don't know how to be honest with ourselves. It takes a crisis to break the external shell we've constructed for society. When that shell breaks and the emotions spill out, we're shocked. Where did all this come from?

Since my external shell began to crack, I've become very vulnerable, particularly to my mother and Larry. They have always hurt me, and they still continue to hurt me. They say things like, "You're smart, you can cure yourself." That's their encouragement since they found out I have AIDS. Whenever they make a comment that hurts, I become defensively aggressive, and I no longer have the energy for such battles. I no longer want to find myself reacting aggressively. And I don't want to waste time on people who hurt me.

Four years ago, soon after Kevin died, Larry put his arms around me and wanted to kiss me. I said, "No." He didn't insist. I felt he wanted to take advantage of me when I was weak and down. He didn't respect what I had been through. I said nothing about it to my mother. I didn't want to make a scene. I needed them to take care of Justin from time to time. I needed them to help me financially. I had no one else. Larry was still there for me, even after I had pushed him away. And I couldn't afford to get depressed because of what he had done. My own survival was more important, and if I needed him to ensure my survival, I was going to put aside his indiscretion and use him for my own ends.

But, as I've discovered, there's a price to pay for their help because it doesn't come with an open heart. They're constantly reminding me of all they've done for me. And somehow this reminder feels like emotional blackmail. Recently, since I haven't been following their advice, they've been refusing to take care of Justin.

I wanted to work with women who are HIV positive and had AIDS. Certain organizations have approached me to speak for them, to participate in decision-making. I've already traveled to several cities to speak to women who have the virus. And they have refused to take care of Justin when I had to go away. My mother wants me to be home in bed all the time. She continually says, "You have to conserve your energy." They don't want me to be active in the organization. Larry doesn't want to see me being independent. He likes to have control. He feels good when putting others down. And I see I can no longer count on him. Now, when I go away, I find someone else to take care of Justin. Which means I no longer need to see Larry and rarely see my mother.

I have never really had any love for my mother. My relationship with her has always been disappointing in some way. I don't always want to get hurt and then try to get over it. I'm the one who is sick, I'm the one who is going to die. I have no more energy to waste on a relationship that gives me nothing but emotional pain.

Neither my mother nor my sister want to talk about my illness. They don't want me to mention death. They don't want to hear that I'm tired. When I told my sister I had AIDS, I had hoped it would bring us closer together. It didn't work out that way. She's clearly not interested in having a relationship with me.

As we were growing up, whenever my sister and I fought, my mother always said, "Joan is right." Or, "Dianne is right." One of us was right and the other was wrong. That created a great deal of animosity between us. There was always blame, never encouragement. And that's how my sister raises her children. As a result, they are always fighting, both physically and verbally. Isabel and Justin also fight a great deal. Children take after their parents. Perhaps my aggressivity and anger influences the way they act with each other. I'm trying to understand what I need to do as a mother if I want my children to grow up to be balanced individuals. I pay attention to how I act around them and how they react to me and to each other. Now if I see them fighting, I take them in my arms, kiss them, and tell them I love them. And they feel my words. They see that I love them equally. It's like a miracle how their behaviour changes.

The decision when to tell Isabel about my condition was a difficult one. Last summer she said, "Mom, I know you're sick, but I don't know the name of your illness." I didn't answer. I didn't want to lie, and I wasn't ready to tell her what I had.

I often speak in schools, where I'm regularly asked if my daughter knows about my condition. I say, "No." They ask me, "Why?" I tell them that I think she's too young. When I was diagnosed, she was only six. But recently I've found myself talking to girls who are twelve, and my daughter is going to be eleven soon. At the end of one talk I gave, a girl of fifteen came up to me.

She said, "My father died of AIDS three years ago, and I found out he had AIDS two weeks before he died. It was painful to have him die, but knowing that people hid his condition from me made it worse. No one told me what was going on. I would have liked to know that he had AIDS and didn't have very much time to live. I would have liked the opportunity to get closer to him, to know him better."

She added, "I'm still angry that no one told me about his illness before." She was very nervous talking to me, and I was very moved. She finished by saying, "I told you this thinking my experience might help you with your daughter." Since she was twelve when her father died, had she known about his condition earlier, she would have had to be at least eleven, if not younger. I compared her situation to Isabel's and thought I didn't want her to blame me for not having told her soon enough.

This girl's story helped me to finally tell her. I realized I hadn't told her, not only to protect her, but also to protect myself. I thought, Here I go again, leaving her. She was only three and a half when I left Peter, and a few years later I tell her, "Your mother has AIDS and will die soon." I was afraid of her tears, afraid of her pain.

I finally told her in Peter's presence. I thought it might be easier for her to have her father there when I broke the news. Peter already knew. I had told him four years ago, and at that time I asked to see Isabel more often, not just during the time allotted by the court. He totally agreed.

I began by saying, "Do you remember, a few weeks ago you asked me about work? You thought I was no longer working, and I said that I was still with the company." She nodded. "I was lying. And I don't feel good about that. You were right, I had stopped working. I'm on a long sick leave."

She looked at me with wide eyes. I said, "I guess you now want to know what I have." She nodded again. I had a tremendous amount of difficulty getting the words out of my mouth. Finally I said, "This is

very hard for me to say because I have AIDS." Then I just br
and cried. Peter was also crying. It was so difficult to break s
to a little girl. I asked her if she knew about AIDS.

She said, "Yes." I asked her if she had any questions.

She asked me if I was going to die.

I said, "I'm not going to die tomorrow, but this illness has no cure."

I didn't say my immune system is very low and I can be sick any
day now. She came over, put her arms around me, and said, "I love
you." And started crying.

I told her what could happen if she told her friends. I said they
might not want to be friends with her anymore, not because they
don't want her as a friend, but because their parents might not allow
them to play with her. The parents might be afraid of this illness
because AIDS has a lot of fear attached to it. I said, "If you say nothing, it'll hurt no one. If you need to talk to someone because you're
worried, you can call me or your grandmother."

She said, "Grandma knows?"

I said, "Yes."

"Auntie Helen knows?"

I said, "Yes."

Then she was upset, "Everyone knew but me!"

She asked me who will take care of Justin. I reassured her. She
knew Ralph and Joyce, and I told her that Justin was going to live
with them.

I had found a family for him fairly early because I don't think a child
can just be transplanted to a new family from one day to the next. I
didn't want him to grow up in my family, so I had to look for
another one willing to adopt him. Also, when I'm sick in hospital, I
need someone to take care of him. If I get pneumonia, I might have
to be in there for a month. I was talking to my social worker and told
her I'd like people to adopt Justin who appreciate nature, are not
violent, are sensitive, spiritual. I gave her a whole list. And she said,
"That sounds very much like a couple I've known for over fifteen
years." A month later, she called to say they would like to meet me.

This couple had tried to have children and couldn't. When I met them, they told me they were hoping to adopt a child. They are wonderful and very generous people. They laugh a lot. They're musicians in a symphony orchestra. Ralph teaches the flute. Joyce teaches piano. They have a heart. If I die tomorrow, I know that in their house Justin will not be abused either physically or psychologically. Also, Justin likes them very much. When they met him, he was already three and a half years old. Now he's going on five.

At first they took him once every two weeks, which was not enough to have him integrated into their daily life. I want their place to be a second home for him. Perhaps I will live another year but I can also become very sick in two weeks and die. This illness is totally unpredictable. I don't want Justin to suddenly find himself at Ralph and Joyce's full time. It would be too much of a shock. Starting next week, he's going to spend three days a week with them. Monday, Tuesday, and Wednesday. This allows him to gradually get accustomed to them and their place. It's a delicate situation because I'm not dead yet. But I want them to be my son's parents when I die, and I need to ease him into that reality for when it will happen. I cannot think of Justin in terms of years anymore.

The last time I was in hospital, I realized that if Justin goes to school near where I live, which is what I want, and I become ill, I won't be able to pick him up, and he won't be able to come home because someone else will be taking care of him. What will happen to school? Ralph and Joyce are an hour and a half away from me. I expressed my concern to Joyce when she visited me in the hospital, and she suggested that Justin enrol in a private school near their house. They offered to pay for it. I was faced with the same situation I had with my daughter. I have never been in touch with Isabel's school. I have never helped her with her homework. And I've missed that. Now, I won't be able to follow Justin's schoolwork. And is he soon going to be at Joyce and Ralph's the whole week? But if I want a solid future for my son, this is what needs to be done.

I would prefer to lose Justin while I'm still alive, knowing he's going to be in a good home. I would prefer to see him with Ralph and Joyce, rather than having him beside me till I die. Then he would be put into a foster home, with foster parents I wouldn't know and who might abuse him. At least this way I know who will adopt him, and I know he will have a secure future with them. For that, I have to be willing to let him go before I die. Having made that decision, which was tremendously difficult, I proved to myself that I was capable of love.

I will soon make a video cassette for my son and daughter where I will speak to them. The video will be for when they're fifteen or eighteen. I will tell them I know what it's like to be that age, and it's a difficult time. I'll talk to them about my philosophy of life. I'll tell them I love them, and I'll always be there for them. And I know I will always be in their hearts.

I've been seeing the psychologist for three years now. First, two years with a group, and then individually. One clue to how much I've changed during that time is the people I now have around me. The people I'm meeting these days are truly good human beings. Two women I met in the group are now my best friends. We have the same fears. When we're together, we allow each other to talk about suffering and death. We listen to each other. One will talk of suicide, and the other will say, "I know exactly what you mean." She might not really be thinking about suicide seriously, but she needs to talk about it. She needs to say, I'm terrified of seeing myself physically disintegrate. We can verbalize these fears without being afraid that the other will say, "You shouldn't talk like that." You can't always keep quiet, be strong, and pretend everything is fine when it's not.

Before, whenever someone asked me how I was, I always said, "Terrific!" And it wasn't true. I had a headache. I was tired. I was angry. But I always said I was fine, more than fine, great. Before, I never wanted to talk about myself. I only wanted to talk about things that were pleasant, amusing, fun. Four years ago, I would never have revealed anything about my private life. Now, when someone asks me how I am, I can say, "I'm a little tired."

Recently I was feeling very depressed, and I actually picked up the phone and called a friend. I cried and he offered to come over. I said, "No, no." Then I said, "Well, if you don't mind, come."

Normally, I would have washed my face, applied makeup. This time I didn't do anything. I allowed him to see me as I was, a tear-stained face, red and swollen, going to pieces. And it helped me to allow myself to be vulnerable, to actively seek affection and comfort.

I had circulated a letter inviting women who were HIV positive or had AIDS to call me, to exchange experiences, views, ideas to help ourselves and each other. In the letter, I told them when I was diagnosed and where I was having difficulties finding help. Some women called me. One of the women who called was Lynn, and we got along very well. She lived out of town, and when she had to come in for some tests and treatments, I told her she was welcome to stay here.

She stayed with me for a week. That was quite a learning experience. The virus is just one of many illnesses she's had all her life. She got spina bifida when she was young. She has had seventeen operations for it, and she's only thirty-three. A nerve was cut in her back, and this affected her legs. She can no longer straighten her toes and walks with her toes curled in. She needs special shoes. Yet she's full of energy, never complains, and still has the capacity to enjoy life. She also had a colostomy and has a bag on her stomach for the elimination of waste. She has fought all her life and considers these physical problems as simply a part of living.

A few days after she left, I became ill and had to go into hospital. While there, I met a young woman who had open ulcers on her legs and had to have bandages up to her thigh. She couldn't walk. She had to be given a bath every morning with a certain medication that was extremely painful. Yet she could still smile.

Both Lynn and the girl in the hospital have known a tremendous amount of physical suffering, yet still continue. And they live with a positive attitude. They're not saying, I'm going to take a pill and finish my life because I can't take this anymore. They're suffering all the time and still have a desire to live. They're fighters.

As a result of my contact with such people, I'm evolving in my attitude toward suffering. Two years ago, I would have refused to suffer for one week. I planned to take my life into my own hands.

Four years ago, I wanted to commit suicide. These days, I'm finding that my limit of acceptable suffering is changing. My psychological tolerance in the face of suffering is widening.

But the last time I was in hospital I was overcome by the suffering around me. Someone down the hall, who also had AIDS, was delirious, yelling and crying throughout the day and night. Why? What is the purpose of such suffering? I need to believe that suffering does give something to people, otherwise it makes no sense. But in the hospital, I fell into a panic. I felt powerless. When I finally got out of there, I wanted to regain control of my life and had two rooms of the house repainted. That was something I could control, the colour of the walls.

When I'm calm, I believe suffering can stretch people's limits. Vaccines have been invented because people have suffered. Medicine was born in response to people's suffering. Revolutions have been fought to put an end to social injustice and human misery. Suffering has helped to better the human condition. It has been a catalyst to push us beyond our limits. Maybe suffering isn't necessary, but, both on a physical and psychological level, it has always helped people to evolve.

I believe the pain of my past has made me stronger. And healing the past can help me to die better. If you have not healed your life, if you have never faced obstacles, then dying must be very frightening.

When I was young, I used to ask an external force to help me in time of difficulties. Now I believe in myself, as if this external force is now within me. Recently I've noticed that, as my anger has been diminishing, this inner force has become stronger. And a dream I had in my early twenties keeps coming back to me. I was sleeping on a table outside, and I woke up in my dream, very worried. "What am I doing on this table?" I didn't have a cover over me, and I was cold. In my head I heard a voice say, "Don't worry, we'll take care of you." There was such love and calm in that voice. When I heard it, I felt a total, encompassing love around me. I was no longer worried and went back to sleep. I've never forgotten that dream. Every time something difficult happened to me, I remembered that voice. When I feel a love within, it is like the love I felt in that voice. But where did that voice come from? Did it come from within?

These days, I feel this inner force is so strong that I can strengthen my immune system. I believe I can cure myself. But would I have the desire to do so? I don't know.

I have an immense curiosity to know what's after death. I've always felt a tremendous nostalgia for that other world, up there. A yearning, as if I've lost something and now I'm on the verge of remembering what I've lost. Since I've been young, my goal has always been to understand the purpose of this world. Why have human beings been created? Why does suffering exist? Why joy? Why wealth? Why poverty? When I know the answer, I will have attained my goal.

At an early age, I sensed there was a depth to existence that was not evident and could not be seen by the naked eye. For me, death has never been something to fear. And now death will be a deliverance. Something beautiful. Why? Why? Is it because I've never really been happy in this life? Now, here I am with an illness that's taking me toward death, and for the first time I love life. I love. I love life and I love death. Now I must choose.

I've come to a crossroads. If I let myself go, I will know what I've always wanted to know. Though I love my daughter and my son, I would at last return to what I've longed for but could never name because I had forgotten what it was. This enormous desire will finally be fulfilled. And that's very attractive. What will it take for me to stay here and live? I have children, I love them. But this call from the unknown is so much stronger. What is that? Maybe I'm looking for a love I have never experienced here on earth. I know my children love me. I love them. But that's not fully enough for me. I want love with a capital L. That great, enormous love. I'm looking for that love I feel within when I touch my inner force. I would like to meet that love outside of myself. To feel that people have the capacity to love with such power and strength. That perfect, pure love.

I do believe one needs to be ready to receive the full force of such tremendous love. A terminal illness gives one time to prepare. And it gives one an opportunity to grow and open, then die in peace, ready to receive. Illness is a hard vehicle for growth, but sometimes that's what it takes.

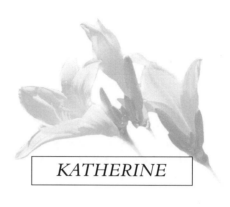

KATHERINE

A doctor at the palliative care unit gave me Katherine's name, saying she would enjoy being interviewed. At sixty-eight and suffering from terminal cancer, she would be willing to look at her death. She had no fear of the end.

Katherine enthusiastically welcomed me from her hospital bed in a spacious private room. She was vivacious and excited about discussing her views on life. She truly enjoyed talking. To her, everything was worth examining carefully, everything mattered. The first time we met, she didn't allow me to turn on the tape recorder. She first insisted on asking me questions about why I wanted to write this book. She wanted to know what else I had written, and I brought a copy of my last book, In Search of Paradise, *to our next meeting.*

Our third and last meeting was close to Christmas, and she asked if we could continue after the New Year because a number of friends wanted to visit her, and she had to conserve her energy. I understood, but I was concerned. I called the doctor who had given me her name and jokingly asked her to make sure Katherine would be alive then because she was so exceptional.

Katherine died before the New Year. I felt terrible, but after thinking long and hard, I decided to include what she told me, as incomplete as it was.

A few months later, Katherine's cousin called me to say he had the

book I had lent her; could he give it back to me? When he arrived
with the book we talked for a few minutes. He told me that Katherine
had been an alcoholic. That gave me a shock. She had never mentioned
this. But we had talked only three times, and only two of the inter-
views dealt with her life. I reasoned that this might have come out
with more interviews. Surely she must have stopped drinking, at least
when she was admitted to hospital the last time, if not after her earlier
jaw and sinus operation.

What finally stayed with me was how I saw her last, when she was
definitely happy, delighted, fully aware, as if ready to go on a surprise
trip. As she said, "I don't want to miss anything."

Illness doesn't happen from one day to the next. It's like a creative
idea. It needs time to germinate. The seed often comes from an
unknown source, such as an internal reaction triggered by an external
event which is later forgotten. The seed then settles in the soil of the
subconscious. At this point, if it doesn't find itself in fertile soil, it is
unable to bear fruit. If it does encounter fertile ground, it begins to
sprout roots and in time blossoms. This illness first appeared as a
cold, certainly after it had already spent a fair amount of time
germinating. Now, nearly three years later, I have terminal cancer.

The cancer started with the uvula, the little handle that hangs
down in the middle of the throat, just above the back of the tongue.
You can see it when you open your mouth. Two years ago I had an
operation to remove it.

The operation clearly did not stop the progress of the cancer,
which continued to work its way to my jaw and sinus bone. The
doctor who had operated on the uvula sent me to another surgeon,
supposedly one of the best in the field.

Before I agreed to the operation, I had a serious talk with him and
made it clear I didn't want to be his guinea pig. I said, "I've already
had one major operation and know the energy required to recuperate. It's no picnic. If this operation will give me a life where I can be
autonomous, walk around, do the things I enjoy, I will agree to go

through it." I wanted to be certain I could have a good quality of life after such an operation. I didn't want to end up simply shuffling from one bed to another. In that case, I would prefer to let the disease follow its natural course without interference.

The doctor said, "You have a very good chance of recovery." He told me there were risks involved and to a certain extent, the operation was a gamble, but he led me to believe I would be fine if I made it. He gave me the impression that there were only two options. Either I would die on the table, or I would be back to normal.

I gave my consent. Last June, both jawbones were removed as well as part of the sinus bone. Three weeks after the operation I was sent home, even though I was still very weak. I was told I would recover faster in a familiar environment. Conceptually that sounds like a wonderful idea, but I was living alone. I didn't have anyone to take care of me, and I could hardly swallow, which meant I couldn't eat and certainly couldn't recuperate.

At home I found myself degenerating. I went to see the surgeon every week for a routine checkup and he seemed totally unconcerned about my general condition. He was only interested in the result of his handiwork. Whenever he checked my mouth, he went into a fit of ecstasy. "It's beautiful, beautiful, beautiful. We did a marvellous job."

I said, "But doctor, I can't drink, I can't eat. I'm getting weaker by the day. I'm dying."

He said, "No, no, you're exaggerating. You're fine. That you even made it through such a complex operation proves your heart is very strong. You're as solid as a rock. And the work inside your mouth is magnificent, worthy of an illustration in a medical book."

My cousin, who regularly drove me to the appointments, said, "Your doctor's enthusiasm is certainly reassuring." I wasn't so convinced.

Though I had visitors, most of the time I was alone in the house. I had difficulty moving around. I had heart palpitations, plus I was very weak. I couldn't eat. I could barely drink. It took me two hours of constant sipping to finish one can of Ensure because it was so hard for me to swallow. I was getting weaker and weaker, and the doctor kept saying, "You're fine. Everything is perfect. You simply need the will to drink. You have to want to drink. The difficulty is in your mind."

I said, "Don't you think the problem might be physical? Half my throat is blocked as a result of the operation. It takes forever till the liquid goes down."

The surgeon wasn't interested in what I was saying. According to him, I wasn't drinking because I didn't want to cooperate. He wanted me to drink eight cans of Ensure a day, and it took me two hours to drink one. Two hours of constant, laborious work, little sips at a time. It was totally exhausting. I kept telling myself, "You have to finish it. You have to finish it." I felt like I was going to be sipping Ensure forever, to eternity.

We each have our own private little hell into which we wander by accident. Once there, we realize there is no escape. Like Sartre's *No Exit*. I felt I had made a terrible mistake, and now here I was sipping away bravely with no reprieve. Punishment for my error. Needless to say, I was not happy.

My weekly appointment with the surgeon became a biweekly and then a monthly appointment. He felt there was no reason for me to see him more often. He said the only obstacle to my improvement was my unwillingness to drink. I believed him. He was the specialist. He should know. What did I know about such things?

Time passed. My condition continued to deteriorate. I began to have diarrhea. The moment I took a sip of either water or Ensure, I had to run for the toilet. As I grew weaker and weaker, I couldn't run. I could barely drag myself to the toilet. Can you imagine? Then I had to try to clean up the mess. That took forever, plus I was constantly nauseous because I was so weak. It was torture.

I had an appointment with the surgeon for the beginning of November, and by the eighth of October I couldn't stand up. I was in a state of panic. The word isn't encompassing enough to fully describe how I felt. I was drowning. I was struggling for air while my strength was ebbing away. I was grasping for life. In desperation I put an SOS call through to the doctor's secretary and said, "I must see him today. I can't wait till November. I'm not going to be alive by then."

She must have thought I was exaggerating. She replied in a very calm and authoritative voice, "He's away till the end of the month."

I said, "I can't wait that long. He must have an assistant for emergencies."

"No. You'll have to see your GP."

"But my GP is not a surgeon. He knows nothing about this operation."

"That's all I can do," she said.

Sometimes you wonder why there are murders. For the first time in my life, though I felt weak, I felt a tremendous surge of anger. I hate to think what would have happened had I been able to act upon it. I then called the doctor who had operated on me the first time, on the uvula. He is a wonderful, caring man. I had wanted him to do the operation on my jaw and sinus, but he said I needed a specialist for such an operation. That wasn't his field. He did say if there were any problems, or if I didn't understand something, I was free to contact him, and he would do whatever possible to help.

I called him. His secretary immediately pulled out my file and said, "Go to emergency. I'll tell the doctor about you, and he will be there sometime today."

I said, "This can't wait, nor can I take a taxi. I can't walk. I would need an ambulance." I was crying. Needless to say, I wasn't myself. I've always been an independent person. It was always I who helped other people, not the other way around. Finding myself in such a vulnerable position was quite confusing.

The secretary said, "Calm down a little, pack a few necessities into a little bag, and call somebody you know to help you. Be at the hospital for two o'clock. The doctor will be there."

It was already eleven. I called my cousin, who immediately came, packed a bag for me and virtually carried me in his arms to the car. We arrived in the hospital for two, and the nurses were already waiting for me. The doctor was there within minutes. As soon as he saw the condition I was in, he called to the nurse and asked for a room, fast.

I was immediately taken to a room, where he examined me. By this time I was in terrible pain and losing consciousness. I was given morphine for the pain. The next day, they inserted a small tube through my nose which was guided down to my stomach. Then they cut a small opening on my stomach, through which the tube was pushed out, and then it was attached to an outside feeding tube. Then they pulled out the one from my nose. Or something like that. Now I have a tiny opening on my stomach, and the feeding tube goes into this opening. It is through this tube that I receive the daily food I need. I no longer have to force myself to drink anything. What a relief.

I was admitted on Tuesday. Had the feeding tube installed on Wednesday. On Friday I came to, meaning I actually felt alive. The following week, a nurse told me they hadn't expected me to survive the weekend.

At first the doctor came to see me three or four times a day. Not like the doctor who had operated on my jaw and sinus bone. I never heard from him again. When I came back to life, my doctor said, "I have good news and bad news." He was laughing. We have a close relationship and can joke around, tease each other. "The good news is that everything is perfect, your heart is excellent, your stomach, kidneys, liver, intestines, lungs are all in perfect working order. But," he continued, "when we put down the tube we saw evidence of cancer down your throat."

I quickly said, "I don't want another operation."

"Unfortunately, we couldn't operate now anyway because you're too weak. Maybe later."

I was absolutely adamant. Calm but firm. "I don't want to hear about another operation. First the uvula had to be taken out, then my jaw and sinus bone, what next and when will it stop? There is only so much I can take."

He said, "You're right, I agree with you. We could give you radio-therapy."

"No. Don't even mention that word."

The radio I received after the first operation was partially responsible for the problem I had swallowing after the second operation. The radio had made my throat very dry, it had burnt my saliva glands. Nothing went down my throat because I had no saliva. I never realized how important saliva was, to talk, to eat. After the first operation, the doctor said, "I don't like radiotherapy, but you have so many chances on your side that we really have to give it a try."

I was operated on in February, and one morning in June I woke with a terrible sore throat. I went to the bathroom mirror and saw that my whole neck was swollen. By night I looked like I had a rubber tire around my neck. My body looked monstrous. I looked ready to join the circus. The swelling was so enormous I couldn't bend my head. Plus it was painful. My lips had become enormous. They protruded several inches. I looked like a Masai warrior with a huge lip disk.

When I went to see the doctor, he said, "We're lucky we didn't have anything till now. The swelling is a reaction to the radio. Believe me, it will disappear, but I can't say when."

It took three months. By the time the swelling went down, I had stopped the radio.

I told my doctor, "I refuse to play with radiotherapy again. If, after all I've been through, there is still cancer, it means my time is due. We all have to go."

The doctor said, "Yes, but I'd like you to be positive."

"How much more positive can I be? I've had two operations for cancer. Now there is something else. Why try to fight like Don Quixote with the windmills? Clearly, I'll never get better. Leave me in peace, and when the time comes, I want to go in a dignified way. I want to see straight and pay attention to where I'm going. All I ask is for you to help me with the pain. Other than that, I don't want to be drugged, and I don't want any distractions like miraculous efforts to save me. At this point one more operation or one more session of radio is simply a distraction. These procedures create fear and make you feel like a caged animal. Instead of concentrating on what is happening, that you're dying, you are diverted by stupid reactions. Just help me with the pain, and I'll make out my will."

He was surprised. "I didn't expect you to talk this way. But I respect your wishes. In some cases we can't take all the pain away, but we'll do the best we can."

The next day I was transferred to this room on the palliative care unit. My pain is now under control, as much as possible. For the time being, I'm not suffering at all, and I'm fully conscious. Exactly what I want right to the end.

It's important to pay attention when you feel your time has come and you're ready to die. I want to be there when it happens. I want to know what's going on. When I go to a concert or read a book or talk to somebody, I am fully there. I'm focused on the event at hand. Why would it be any different for dying?

Even while I was throwing up at home or trying to get to the bathroom, I was amazed at how my body functioned. From time to time I was able to remove myself from the pain and discomfort and simply watch the movements of my body. It was fantastic. When I was well, I would sometimes go for a walk and think, My legs are moving through the air. They're moving one after the other, like in a graceful dance. My muscles are all coordinated. It was magic.

I definitely want to be there to see how this body will stop functioning. When this beauty and grace will no longer be, what will happen? When the magic of this body vanishes, will it then be replaced by another sort of magic? It's easy to miss your own death, and then you might also miss the beginning of a new magic. I don't want to miss anything.

When I was in pain, I wasn't thinking of dying, I was just concerned with the pain. My whole attention was focused on it. And that's extremely narrow. I feel when you are about to witness your own death you need as wide a vision as possible. You can only achieve that if you're relaxed and calm.

At the moment, I'm simply waiting for the curtain to rise, for the play to begin. Though I have found serenity and tremendous generosity here in the hospital, I don't call this living, not for me. The nurses are treating me like a baby. I can enjoy that for a few days, but I'm an adult, and being treated like a baby makes me feel diminished. I want to be able to get up and walk on my own two feet. But I can't. I don't even have enough energy to stand up. I can't get out of bed alone. I need help to go to the bathroom.

C03

Now I can better understand what my mother must have lived through. She was ill for twenty years with deforming arthritis. Every year her condition grew worse and worse, more and more debilitating. She was in constant pain. Every single joint ached. Every morning my father had to move her from the bed to the wheelchair. That changes your perspective over time. My illness is too recent. There hasn't been enough time for my outlook on life to change. Not like my mother. Over the years, her vision grew smaller and smaller. Pain can do that. Pain is like a small child constantly screaming for attention. The last year she fell in the house and broke her hip. By then she was so weak she could hardly do anything for herself.

She didn't want to be selfish, but I was her only child. She needed me and I wanted to be there for her. Mind you, she was a nuisance, but that was an understandable weakness given her situation.

As her condition progressed from bad to worse, with emergencies happening virtually every week, I regretted not ever having had a sister or brother. I had to bear the full burden of my mother alone. I had no siblings to help. When my mother was at the hospital, I went every night to see her. My father worked long hours, and he relied on me to be there for her. He did what he could, but he felt quite helpless. Emotionally it was difficult for him. Though I loved my mother, at times it was certainly trying, and I was left wishing I had had a different life.

My mother wanted me to get married, have children, but you have no idea how ill she was, how much she suffered. I couldn't leave her. She never stopped me. She would have loved to see me marry and come home with grandchildren, but she didn't realize how much she needed me. I was the one to give her a bath every morning. I did all the grocery shopping. If I left, who would take care of her needs?

Several times I almost got married but broke off the engagement before reaching the altar. How can you put such a heavy load on a young man's shoulders? He is trying to build a career and can't be preoccupied with a sick mother-in-law. Who knows, my husband might be transferred to another city for work. How could I follow him? There was no way. The last few years, my mother needed constant attention. She had to be taken to the hospital for cortisone shots. I knew that any time of day or night I might be called home. I never knew what to expect. There were days when she had to be rushed to the hospital, in pain, screaming. And it was expensive. In those days we didn't have health care or health insurance. You even had to pay for your own toilet paper. It cost a fortune. I had to help out financially because my father didn't make very much. He was a meek, gentle man.

What's the use of thinking it might have been different? It's all over now.

Martha was my best friend from the time we met at school. She had known my mother and had known what I had to go through. She was the only one with whom I discussed my situation. We talked about the pros and cons of getting married. Was it possible to be there for my husband as well as my mother? She, too, was going through trying times with her family. A younger brother had committed suicide. She had had a heartbreaking love affair and as a result never married, either.

Two years ago, Martha died of breast cancer. By then my own cancer had also been diagnosed, so it seemed we were going through the same predicament. We exchanged views on therapy. Doctors. I had thirty sessions of radio and she had thirty-nine. They gave her the radio through her arm to her breast, and her arm started to swell. Near the end, the top part of her arm was the colour of an eggplant. Plus it was huge. It was so swollen she had to wear a sling around her neck to carry her arm. She was in terrible pain. She asked the doctor what he could do. He suggested amputating the arm. I said to her, "Martha, an amputation isn't going to cure your cancer."

But she said to the doctor, "Do it. I refuse to let the cancer get me."

In the end, the doctor decided against it because she was getting weaker and weaker, till finally she had to be sent to the hospital. Within weeks, she was transferred to the palliative care unit. She was put in a room with four beds, plus one in the centre because they had no more space.

For me, privacy is essential, essential. If you're in pain, you can't be nice to your neighbours. You can't be polite. There is no such thing as quietly screaming when you're in pain. Also, the nurses come in the middle of the night to give a patient an injection or medication, and they have to put on the light. Or, after an operation, a patient returns to the room at four in the morning. There's no peace.

The day after I finally came back to normal, I looked around me to realize I had been placed in a private room. My dream! And I hadn't even asked for a private room. I would think when people are terminal they would want to be alone. I certainly do. That's not the time to socialize.

I would like to reflect in peace and quiet while waiting for the end. I would like to remember what I've most enjoyed about life. Like the beauty I've encountered. Anything can be beautiful, a piece of music, a tiny flower, someone's eyes, a strip of cloth. I've always had an appreciation for beauty. This is not something you can learn, you're born with it. When I was a little girl, even before I went to school, I had a collection of lovely ribbons. Only recently did I throw them away. Some were embroidered with metallic threads, others had different textures of velvet or silk. They were colourful little ribbons, nothing grand, but to me they were beautiful. As a decorator, whenever I touched fine fabrics, the pleasure I derived was equivalent to the delight I experienced when sipping good wine. I so loved the variety of textures, the subtlety of colours. It was wonderfully inspiring.

I was an interior designer. I did stage designs, costumes, window displays, private homes, schools, offices, stores. Everything. I had my own business, a one-person company. I did well. I started just after the war, and at that time this business was still new, like brie — we had never tasted brie before the war because it was not exported. I started at twenty and only stopped four or five years ago because I wasn't feeling well. At that point, I still had a few select customers. But I couldn't take on anyone new. I was no longer able to run around as I once did.

I had studied art at the École des Beaux Arts at the Museum of Fine Art in Montreal and realized I didn't have as much to say as Matisse, Cézanne, or Gaugin. Also, I had to earn a living. But I enjoyed art tremendously. Whenever I had free time, I went to the museum to linger amongst the paintings and sculptures. I enjoyed the juxtaposition of colours, shapes, textures. The museum was a rarefied atmosphere where the canvases evoked feelings, thoughts, ideas, even memories. Sometimes they gave you a totally new perspective on reality.

Originally I wanted to go to university and become a journalist. I grew very fast, then suddenly stopped, and it was hard on my system. The doctor suggested I stay home for a year to rest. My mother said to him, "If she stays home, she'll go crazy, she's too active." She went to the high school I had attended to talk to one of my teachers, who recommended that she send me to the Beaux Arts at the museum for half days. The teacher said I had an aptitude for art and would enjoy it. Later I could go to university.

When I started at the Beaux Arts, a whole new world opened up to me. In those days all I knew was calendar art. Art school introduced me to the world of fine art. There I was flipping through art books I hadn't even known existed. I discovered classicism, impressionism, expressionism, surrealism. The role of mythology in art. The role of religion. Symbolism. The evolution of the concept of light. A veritable treasure trove! It was fantastic. Up to that time my world had been quite limited. Though I had enjoyed beautiful flowers and ribbons, now I discovered there were people who had devoted their whole lives to art, to the search for the right colour, the right vision, style. People who had spent their whole life on aesthetics.

Had my family's financial situation been more favourable, I would have liked to paint. It wasn't so much that I didn't have as much to say as Gaugin or Cézanne, it was more because I couldn't afford to spend time developing ideas, experimenting with style. To be an artist, you have to have the freedom to devote yourself to your art. I didn't have that luxury. I needed to earn money.

When I discovered I could work with colour and texture as a decorator, I went to study drafting at night. I finished the Beaux Arts at twenty and began as an assistant decorator at Morgan's. Back then, Morgan's was the most elegant department store. There were doormen. The decorator's studio had exquisite decorators. Only millionaires engaged their services.

I wanted to design my own furniture. In those days, there was nothing on the market, there were no furniture manufacturers in North America. At the end of the war, all the factories in the States were still busy with armament production. If you wanted a chair, you had to first design it, then give the drawing to a cabinetmaker. I could never show a customer a specific chair or table. All I could show was a drawing, with small samples of cloth for the covering of chair cushions. Actually, I was selling a piece of paper with bits of fabric glued next to the design. Then, if the customer approved the drawing, I worked with cabinetmakers who made my ideas a reality. Seeing a cabinetmaker begin work on a table or chair that was a mere drawing and then following that piece of furniture to its gradual completion was fascinating. I saw my one-dimensional drawing come to life in three-dimensional space. It was magic.

Not only did I work with interior space, I also consulted on exterior space. Architects experimented with new designs for buildings. Decorators experimented with the look and shape of furniture. It was an exciting time. I had the best years.

I stayed as an assistant at Morgan's for about two years and quickly realized that as a decorator it would be impossible to work with a partner. You couldn't mix two tastes. I wanted to have full control over the style and look of a house. As an assistant, I was helping another decorator and had to follow his taste. I could do no more than make suggestions. I wanted to be responsible for the mistakes. I also wanted to enjoy the successes.

From one day to the next, I left Morgan's and went out on my own. It was a risky move. I had no money, my parents couldn't help me. But it was clear that, if I wanted to move in a specific direction, I had no other choice. Once I started on my own, I was working twenty-four hours a day, enjoying every minute of it.

Soon after I started my own business my mother became very ill. Since I didn't have to be at work for a fixed amount of time, I didn't have a fixed job, she thought I had all the time in the world. She saw me drafting at home and thought that since I was there, I was available. And because she was so ill, she was very demanding. She always wanted me to do little things for her. She didn't understand I had work to do. I had clients to see. I had drawings to complete. Since I had to spend so much time with my mother, I couldn't complete drawings on time. My work slowed down, and as a result I wasn't making enough money. I had no choice but to temporarily give up my own business. I found a job at Simpson's as a decorator. As soon as I had a permanent job, my mother understood and readily accepted that I wouldn't be home before supper. I was working outside of the house, and that she could understand. She just couldn't understand that I would be at home working. It was a foreign concept to her. If I was home I was available. A person who is as ill as she didn't have a realistic perception of reality.

I lived at home till I was thirty-five, till my mother died. Mind you, when I started working at Simpson's, I got my own flat next door. We were living in an apartment building, and at a certain point the apartment next door became free and I moved in. It was a compromise. At least this way I had a semblance of a private life. I could have some privacy.

Even living next door sometimes felt like I was still living with them. I was over there most of the time. I had supper with them. If in the middle of the night there was a crisis, my father came to knock on my door. Sometimes it was a little embarrassing, since I wasn't always alone.

I couldn't possibly leave her to get married and move away, even though I very much wanted children. After my mother died, I once more began to work as a decorator on my own, with my own company, and then somehow there was no time to think about having a family. As the years passed, my desire for children faded. I enjoyed my work and couldn't see myself being responsible for a family. I kept postponing the decision to get married till finally it was too late. Very often I felt, How I would love to lead a normal life, with a husband, lovely children, a decent income. But it has always seemed like an unattainable ideal. Over the years, from time to time, I did miss not having children, but it had to be done. There was no choice.

When I was little, I wanted numerous children because it's very frustrating to be alone, although it builds character. I was lucky to have had lots of friends. My home was where everything happened because one friend's mother wouldn't like us to dirty the living room, another friend's parents didn't like us to play music past eleven, there were always restrictions. At my home we were free. My parents didn't have rigid rules. They enjoyed seeing my friends at the house. Later, when I was older and already living in my own apartment, even though mother was in bed next door, the night was mine. I was free to have friends over, to have parties. Actually, I was rarely alone. I always had good friends with whom I could share ideas and enthusiasms.

After my mother died I quit Simpson's and went back to being an independent decorator. Almost from the day I went out on my own, the business mushroomed. For instance, I decorated a young couple's house. A few years later, I did their nursery. They recommended me to their neighbours and their uncles. I did a house for a couple where the husband was a doctor. He asked me to do his office. Over the years I have dealt with some wonderful people and have followed their lives for decades. As time went on, I would update certain rooms. When their children got married, I was asked to decorate their first home. I was invited to their parties. My customers were like my family. Up to five years ago, I was still dealing with some of my first customers' children.

I loved the work. There was such variety. No two days were the same. And I have dealt with some wonderful people. Decorating was about aesthetics, taste, refinement and the people appreciated the beauty you brought into their home. There was certainly a business element, but the creative side was much more important.

Now it's over. Now I don't even have the strength to move a chair in this room from one corner to another. Nor do I want to. I have spent my whole life decorating, drawing, creating, and now here I am. Quiet. Calm. Something I have very rarely experienced in my life. Now that my pain is under control and my body is no longer demanding my attention, I can appreciate the serene tranquility that has descended upon me.

But I certainly would not call my present state living. To me, living means to be able to walk on your own, eat and drink on your own, and be conscious of your thoughts. I'm conscious, but consciousness is not enough to qualify for full life. If I'm going to live, I want to enjoy what life has to offer. All its various tastes and smells.

I'm grateful for what I have here. I have good care and am secure in the knowledge that I will never again fall into a state of panic because of the pain. But I definitely feel I'm here waiting for the show to begin. This bed is my seat in the theatre. The curtains will soon rise. The play will commence. And I don't even know what kind of a play it will be. A comedy? A tragedy? Maybe a magic show. Whatever the genre, I plan to fully enjoy it. I expect it will be a glorious experience.

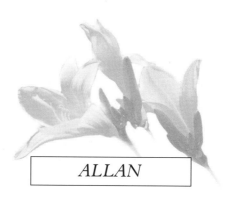

ALLAN

The ALS *Society had given me the name of Allan, a forty-five-year-old poet who would be very willing to talk. I set up our meetings through his brother. Allan's speech was quite difficult to understand because he was already losing control of his vocal cords.*

Interviewing Allan was a very humbling experience. Our first meeting took place at his house. He had a full beard. He was in a wheelchair, but I estimated his height to be about five foot eight, and he was slim. After twenty minutes, he had to go to the bathroom. People with ALS *often have to spend nearly an hour in the bathroom to relieve themselves, waiting for whatever has to come out to do so, since they no longer have control over their muscles. I thought perhaps this was not going to work, taking into consideration his speech difficulty. I waited. I felt I couldn't just leave after a twenty-minute encounter. When he came back, he told me that his wife, who was now dead, had appeared before him in his brother's car after the diagnosis of his illness. He sensed that that detail would hook me, and he was right. From then on, I quickly attuned my ears to the way he talked.*

The second, third, and fourth interviews took place in a hospital to which he had been admitted in an emergency. All subsequent interviews took place in a nursing home, where he had been moved from the hospital. His disease was progressing, he needed constant care, and a home nurse was no longer enough. The nursing home was in the

261

*country, where he had a spacious, private room with sunlight streaming
in through a big window.*

*He complained that the nurses there often could not understand
what he was saying, and he asked me if I had problems. I laughed and
said no. He wondered how that could be. I told him that curiosity
was a big factor.*

*He gave me a copy of his book of poetry at our first meeting, and
during our interviews he launched a second book. Both were self-
published; his son had encouraged him to do this. Since he could not
use his hands, his poems were written down by friends and his son,
when he was available. He was proud to leave his books to his son,
proud to have been able to give voice to his emotions.*

*He had hung up a family picture in his room at the nursing home:
his mother, himself, his two brothers, his son, and a few more people
I didn't recognize, but there was clearly no father. When I inquired
about his father, he asked, "What would you like to know?" His eva-
sion surprised me; he was usually very forthcoming. I asked questions,
groping for something I sensed was important without knowing the
reason. I felt as if I was walking over broken glass. Finally, he told me
his father had committed suicide when he was twenty. It had taken
him four interviews to tell me this. Of course, that shocking event
threw the door wide open for a wider tragedy in Allan's life.*

I regret what I didn't do, not what I did do. Some of the things I did
were very gratifying. But I feel a much greater satisfaction now than
I ever have before in my life. My capacity for pleasure, delight, and
appreciation has bloomed.

Before this illness, I had three large pieces of land. One was a
forest, with eighty trees and a comfortable chalet. I had a country
house by the lake. I owned a house in town. Soon after the diagnosis,
I sold everything. If I were to regain my health, all that acquisition of
property would no longer interest me. I would live with no more
than the bare essentials. I wouldn't even want a car. I would find an
apartment in an area where I could easily walk to stores. And I would

spend my time writing for the pure pleasure of expression. I suppose I could return as a teacher, but I don't know if I would. I would certainly continue to work on my personal evolution, something I've only learned to do since my illness. If I could walk again, regain my health, it would be incredible. In my dreams I see myself healed. In my daydreams I imagine myself healthy. And I would never return to my life as it was before. This illness has taught me how to live.

Now I'm in a nursing home where I'll stay till the end. I would like to leave this life serene and peaceful, not in the midst of a physical catastrophe, choking and fighting for my life. I'd like to leave feeling good about life and good about death. But before my death I have a lot of work to do. Part of that work involves moving toward a full acceptance of my illness. While I could still live at home, I didn't fully accept my diagnosis. I was fighting to live. My illness was a question of adaptation instead of acceptance. As long as my finances allowed me to stay in the apartment with twenty-four-hour-a-day help, I lived my illness, more or less. Here, in the nursing home, I can finally fully acknowledge my illness and accept it. The side effect of this acceptance has been my spiritual growth.

I'm trying to take one day at a time, to live in the present and not look into the future. Also, I'm trying to move closer and closer to a state of serenity. I don't yet have the serenity I need to face my end. When I was still living at home, it was hard for me to work on acceptance and inner peace. There was too much uncertainty and tension. At home, different people looked after me. When a crisis happened, I had to be taken to the hospital, and a few days or weeks later I was again sent back home. The going back and forth was quite stressful. I needed to know there was a constant to my situation. This private room in the nursing home fills the bill. It provides the needed atmosphere. Here, I know I will not be moved. No matter what happens, I can be looked after in my room. The nursing home has all the required personnel right here. Though I liked living at home, the time has come for me to prepare for death.

The progress of the disease is accelerating. I can feel my physical deterioration. I have greater difficulty in chewing and swallowing my food. I have regular fits of choking. My ability to communicate with others has become even more limited. It takes tremendous energy and time to articulate what I need to say, and people have a hard time understanding me. I have no physical strength. My head just drops over my chest if not supported from the back. I sometimes have to get up two or three times a night to go to the toilet, and I have to stay there for about an hour each time. When I sleep, my muscles move involuntarily, which regularly wakes me up. ALS is not a painful illness, but it's very, very uncomfortable and it makes itself very present. It takes energy to eat, to talk, everything. I'm very aware of my body. It's an illness that requires an enormous amount of energy just to live, which means you're almost always in a state of fatigue. Yet I can hardly do anything anymore. I can't move without someone's help. My very life depends on others, and this total dependence can be very frightening.

ALS destroys the motor neurons and the brain's capacity to move the muscles. Since the muscles are not in use, they atrophy. The duration of the illness varies tremendously with each person. But generally life expectancy is anywhere between two and five years after diagnosis. But Stephen Hawking, the physicist, has lived with it for thirty years. Eventually, if you live long enough, the muscles around the lungs also cease. Once the breathing is affected, you're hooked to a machine. I've clearly stated in my will that I don't want a respirator. I don't want to be kept alive by artificial means. What's difficult is not knowing how much time you have left.

This ridiculous situation has forced me to come face to face with myself. And that's not easy. It has pushed me to explore my interior landscape. And it has shown me the importance of inner peace and serenity. Before the illness, I might have thought about serenity on an intellectual level. I certainly never tried to live it. Now I do. The vision of my first wife has been my reference point. That vision has helped me to adjust to my illness, to imbue it with meaning. If I hadn't had that vision, things would have gone very differently.

The illness started four years ago, when I was forty-one. I began to have problems opening the door with my right hand. A month later I went to see my doctor. He referred me to a neurologist, who put me through a series of tests, then asked to see me every three months. He said he had a possible diagnosis but wanted to follow my physical condition for six months to be certain. When I pressed him, he said it could be ALS, but it was too early to tell.

At the time I worked as a teacher with physically and mentally handicapped people and was familiar with certain illnesses. But I knew very little about ALS, popularly known as Lou Gehrig's disease. I began to do research. I noticed a couple of articles in the paper about it, and I wrote away to the ALS Society for information. As time passed and my initial symptoms grew more pronounced, I suspected the doctor was probably right in his initial diagnosis. Still, I was not anxious to have it confirmed.

Seven months after my first visit, he called me in for a meeting. He said he now had all the necessary data for a concrete diagnosis. I was nervous. I asked my brother to come with me to the appointment.

When the doctor gave me the diagnosis, I broke down and cried. Since I had already done my research, he didn't have to tell me much about the illness. I knew the medical profession didn't know how the disease started, and they had no treatment or cure. So I saw no reason to see the neurologist again. Also, I didn't want to be dependent on the medical profession.

My brother drove me home, and I continued to cry in the car. My whole body was shaking. I was in shock. At one point I looked up, and there before me was my wife.

When I was twenty-five, I had a very bad car accident. My wife and five-month-old son were with me in the car. My wife died instantly. And there she stood before me, smiling and surrounded by a brilliant white light which doesn't exist in our physical reality. Such a vision is totally outside of normal experience. I have no idea how long it lasted because I was totally transported to another world. As she stood before me, I felt such a deep well-being. When the vision disappeared, I remember thinking that if I were to die it would be a marvellous experience.

A few days later, the effect of the vision came back, but I couldn't see it. I couldn't take myself back to it. But at least now I know that enormous feeling of well-being can exist. That vision has helped me to continue on, to continue living both mentally and physically. It still carries me. It is the basis of my belief in life. Because of it, I no longer believe in death. Of course, my body will cease to live and I'll be buried, but for me the word death no longer means anything.

Soon after the diagnosis, I quit work because I just couldn't continue anymore physically. I was getting too weak. Alone, at home, I cried a lot. In spite of the vision, I felt a rage against the illness. Why me?

At the time of my diagnosis, my son had just turned seventeen, and it took me a few days to tell him about it. It was very hard to do. How do you tell your teenage son who has already lost his mother that he is now going to lose his father? When I finally got up my courage to talk to him, the first thing he asked was, "Are you going to die?" I couldn't reply. I had such a lump in my throat, I couldn't speak. Nothing came out.

The diagnosis wasn't easy for him. I let him come to me with his questions and I kept him informed about the development of my illness. Also, I discussed Gavin with my two brothers. I didn't want their relationship to change in any way as a result of my condition. They agreed not to treat me with any pity and not to act overprotective toward him. I didn't want my illness to be an emotional burden on him.

As crazy as it sounds, my diagnosis brought Gavin and me closer together. It was positive for our relationship. We did have a good relationship before, but Gavin is a real talker. Before the diagnosis, he had begun to ask all sorts of questions. He came to find me, no matter where I was or what I was doing, to ask questions. I wasn't always prepared to take the time to listen to him or to answer him. After the diagnosis, I was more present for him, which created an intimacy between us that didn't exist before. And I began to appreciate how lucky I was to have a son who was so open, who told me almost everything that happened in his life.

A year later, Gavin went to a CEGEP in another town and lived on campus. Though he came down to see me every weekend, this gave him a physical distance from me which I thought was positive for him. He found a girlfriend and the following year rented his own apartment. When I came to the nursing home, I gave him all my furniture.

In spite of the difficulties and the changes in his life, I think my illness is helping him to mature faster than his age. It's making him more responsible. It's forcing him to think about his future, to be clearer about who he is and where he wants to go. He has applied to go to university next year, and he's busy planning his courses. I'm very pleased about that. If he needs to think about taking care of himself, he has less time to think about me. My illness is not going to prevent him from living his life. I try to minimize my need for him as far as my health is concerned. I try to involve him as little as possible in the logistics of my needs.

When he told me he met a girl he really liked, I was as happy as he was, and it reminded me of myself when I was his age. They were both eighteen when they met, and since she is his first girlfriend, she takes a lot of space in his life. He often talks to me about her and their relationship and freely asks for my opinion and advice. When I was still living in the apartment, he brought her over to introduce me to her. I even wrote a poem about them.

I'm glad he found Melanie. Gavin is an only child. He lost his real mother. And his second mother and I divorced. So his first love relationship is very important. I try to let him know that I take it as seriously as he does. This is his first love and his first sexual contact. I try to make him understand that it's not just a sexual relationship, that the element of friendship is also very important. It doesn't matter how long the relationship lasts, but I would like the experience to be a valuable one for him.

CR

Seeing my deteriorating condition makes him aware of my coming death, and it gives him time to ease into the reality of losing his father. Had I died without any warning, it would have been much harder on him. I know it took him a long time to tell his friends about what was happening to me. Melanie was the first person he told about me. When she introduced him to her parents, the father asked him what I did. He had no choice but to tell him about my condition. The father was the second person he told about me. Later, he told me he had been nervous talking about it. I think now he is more comfortable when someone asks.

Gavin is nineteen now. By the time I die, he will probably be the same age I was when I lost my father. But there the similarities between the two relationships end. I'm there for Gavin when he needs me. I listen to him and he confides in me. I never confided in my father.

My father committed suicide when he was fifty years old and I was twenty. Today he would be seventy-five. He killed himself with a gun. I don't know who found him or how he was found. Either I never knew or I forgot. Frank was four years younger than me, and John was five and a half years younger. They were only sixteen and fourteen and a half when my father died, and we didn't talk about what had happened. They were too young. His suicide was a shock, and I remember crying a lot. At that time, when someone died, the body was on display for three days in the living room. My father was a very sociable man, and a lot of people came to pay their respects. Those three days were like a transition. After his funeral, I simply tried to put the whole thing out of my mind as if it never happened. Only in the last couple of years have I allowed myself to think about him again.

Thinking about him now, I can appreciate the difficulties he had. And I've reached a point where I no longer blame him. But it took me a long time to try to understand his suicide.

CR

My father was the oldest child, and in his time children started to work early and were expected to financially contribute to the household. One day, when he was about twenty-two or twenty-three, his brother arrived home with a girlfriend, and his mother asked him to leave the house to make room for the girlfriend. I think he felt this was a terrible rejection, and he never got over it. When my father got married, he was twenty-nine and my mother was ten years younger than him. At the time, he was working in a warehouse for Canadian Pacific. A few years later, a young man was promoted to a job that rightly should have gone to him. He took this very hard. He quit his job and went to work as a janitor in a bank at nights and began to drink heavily. These two events really affected him, and he couldn't come to terms with them.

My father was almost constantly in a state of depression. Though he was a sociable man who had a lot of friends, now, in retrospect, I can see he wore a mask. This mask hid his depression, his feeling of not being loved, his lack of success at work.

Also, the relationship between my mother and father was very difficult. There was a lot of screaming and fighting. All that noise and animosity scared me. My mother raised us, and my father was absent most of the time. When he was at home, he read the papers. There were always newspapers in the house. I hardly had any contact with him. Except a few days before he died the two of us had a talk. I don't remember what about, but that was the first time we had actually talked.

I felt that my father's suicide was a rejection of me. This was why I had tried so hard to forget about it. You can't just tell people your father committed suicide because then you expose that rejection. I hadn't even told my first wife about him. I told Gavin only when he asked me. I was thirty-seven years old the first time I verbally admitted the circumstances of his death. One day, another teacher and I were talking about death, and he asked how my father had died. It was a casual conversation and a casual question. My answer came out spontaneously, without hesitation. I was surprised. I had held on to that secret for such a long time. It was almost a relief to speak of it openly.

ଔ

I now know that my father was responsible for his actions. I am not to blame for his suicide. Though I didn't figure this out until after I became ill. It's a little odd because the question of responsibility has been a big issue for me most of my life. It has always been important to me. I believe we are responsible for everything we think, say, and do. Those who always blame others for what happens to them are not taking responsibility for their lives. Now I see that my fascination with the question of responsibility has been an inheritance from my father. He had a great deal of difficulty being responsible. I learned by his example how not to be and found a way to be that's better.

Also, my father hid his feelings. This difficulty of facing and dealing with emotions was passed on to his three sons. Now all three of us consciously make an effort to express our emotions. I suppose you can say my father actually left us something of great value. By his example, he showed us how not to be.

I no longer blame him for what he did. Now I would like him to be here so we could learn to talk to each other. I would like to have the chance to talk him out of what he did. I have internal dialogues with him. I talk to him as Gavin's grandfather and ask him to help Gavin. I talk to him about my beliefs, my emotional state, and my physical deterioration. I find it comforting to talk to him. I can feel his support. I feel his presence, and his very presence is his answer to me.

The illness has shown me how to be more sensitive, more open to a larger reality. It has also given me the opportunity to be more intimate with people. I no longer have a need to protect myself. I can discuss my emotional state, my fears, concerns, and pleasures. And my honesty encourages others to reveal themselves on a deeper level. I no longer have superficial exchanges.

Family and friends give me an enormous amount of affection and love. All this warmth was around before the diagnosis, but I was not prepared to accept it. In a relationship, when one person wants to give, the other might not always be prepared to accept because you think, I'll have to give this back at some point. And you're afraid. Accepting something means commitment. Also, accepting something requires a form of communication with the other. Even though we want commitment and contact, we want it without responsibility. If you don't accept anything, you don't need to take responsibility, there is no emotional investment and you can hold onto your illusion of freedom and independence. But this illness has taught me that the person who wants to give does, and that person does not necessarily want something in return. There are people who truly want to give. Your openness to receive their giving is all that's required. This is not easy to do. I've only recently learned to master it.

I'm much more receptive to people now. But I'm also learning that there are different ways to receive. Many friends come and talk to me about their problems. Being there to listen to others makes me feel I'm still alive. I have a use, a reason to live. I can still have an emotional connection to another human being. If I didn't have the capacity to listen, what reason would I have to continue living with such an illness? When people need me, when they discuss their problems with me, it makes me feel part of the human race. In listening to another, I forget about my handicap. The person talking about a problem also forgets about the handicap, they are more preoccupied with themselves than with me.

Physically I'm very diminished, and my situation has allowed me to refine my listening skills. Listening takes tremendous concentration. When people feel you're listening to them, they will confide more and more in you. To listen well, you have to forget yourself during the time that you're listening. After, when you have a comment to make, you can return to yourself. You have to truly listen in the moment and not prepare a response in your head while the other is talking. But when you develop the art of listening, you also have to become responsible for what you hear. This feeling of responsibility grounds me and gives me a deeper sense of connection to the other person. The people who come and confide in me have told me that I present a mirror to them, a mirror which helps them better understand themselves.

The mirror works both ways. In opening myself to listen, I've evolved. But first I had to work at understanding who I was. I needed to understand who was evolving and from what point. And this question of who I was kept changing because physically I was deteriorating, which in turn caused psychological shifts. I had to work at knowing and accepting myself on both a physical and a mental plane. At certain times I have refused to see who I was. From an early age, I developed the skill of disregarding myself. In the past, I have systematically ignored my emotions. This made it virtually impossible for me to be honest with myself.

I grew up believing it was important to control myself and my emotions. This need for self-control was a strong streak in my personality, probably because I saw my father so out of control. Self-control became even more important when acceptance became important. I wanted to be accepted by people outside of the family, people my age. At the beginning of my adolescence, I had a lot of acne and as a result was very shy with girls. I found it hard to ask them out. But I had friends, and we got together in a park near where I lived. These friends were part of a group, and in order for me to be accepted, I developed a very non-aggressive attitude. I created a mask for myself. My own physical development even helped me with this mask.

I began to have acne when I was twelve. At the same time, I also began to have facial hair. The acne made it hard for me to shave. I began with an electric razor, but it didn't do a good job. Then I switched to a regular razor, and I always cut myself. The hair on my face got stronger and stronger, till I had to shave every day. This became very painful because my skin was full of cuts. One day I just let the whole thing grow to a beard. It was more practical than shaving. I got a kick out of having a beard. I experimented with different styles, cut it into different shapes. Having a beard at such a young age, at fifteen, gave me a very distinctive look, it gave me an identity. Shaving it all would have meant giving up a part of myself. My son didn't see me without a beard for the first sixteen years of his life. Three years ago, I cut it. It took me a while to make that decision.

People were so used to seeing me with a beard that the majority said I looked better with it than without. After a while I let it grow out again, partly because I wasn't able to shave due to the illness.

At around age thirteen, when I let my beard grow out, I also started to develop my listening skills because I found it helped me to be accepted. I cultivated my role as the passive listener to ensure my membership in the group. Both boys and girls began to confide in me. They told me about their problems with their girlfriends or boyfriends, problems with their mothers or fathers. They knew I would not make fun of them or judge them. The group needed me, which made me feel validated. I had a role to play. At the same time, I felt responsible for guarding everyone else's pains and hurts. If I would have wanted to be a mediator, I could have resolved some of the arguments in the group because I knew everyone's side, I had everyone's secrets. But I didn't choose to take a more active role. To be a good listener, I had to control my own emotions, sublimate my own feelings. On the odd occasion when I did acknowledge my need to talk and opened up to someone, I felt they weren't really interested in listening to me. I wanted someone to listen the way I listened.

With time and practice, I developed my listening capabilities to such an extent that I was able to totally forget myself and ignore my own needs. When you have ignored yourself for too long, you grow totally incapable of expressing your feelings because you have never developed that skill. And you lose touch with yourself. You don't have a clear sense of direction because you don't know what you want, you never ask yourself.

I was not a very conscientious student. At CEGEP I had studied literature and loved to write. I even wrote several film scripts and did a film at school. But I had no clear idea of what to do with my life. I was interested in teaching but not in academia. All I knew was that I didn't want to work in a place with fixed, rigid ideas and expectations. My philosophy and sociology teachers both suggested I try working with the handicapped. I took their advice but it wasn't a line of work that came from any belief or desire.

I applied as a teacher at a centre for the mentally and physically handicapped. I was accepted and first had to go through a training period. When I began work, I was shocked. I found that the other teachers had emotionally closed themselves off during work and were as handicapped as the people they were supposed to help. They had two faces, one during work and one after. Also, I was surprised to discover that I wasn't as open as I had thought. I had my own prejudices.

I began work with a group of twelve young people, each with a different level of handicap. They varied in age from babies to eighteen year olds. The babies needed a lot of physiotherapy and sensory stimulation. The older ones were taught how to dress, how to eat properly, things that would help them function in society after they left the centre. They also required sensory stimulation but on a more advanced level. Later I worked with smaller groups, which I found more satisfying because I could devote more time to each person.

A few years after I began work, I had the car accident. I felt very guilty about both the accident and my wife's death. At the time of the accident, we had been married eleven months, though we had lived together for three years. She was the first person I had ever loved, and loving another person made me feel safe for the first time in my life. I think my love had a strong element of possessiveness about it. I didn't want to lose this feeling of safety. When I did lose her, I felt as if something had been ripped out of me. The loss happened in such a brutal way.

After the car accident, I was in a semi-coma. I couldn't remember anything for a week. Ten days later, I learned about my wife's death. I was already in shock from the accident, and learning I had lost my wife greatly intensified the pain. Both Gavin and I were in the same hospital, and when we were released, we went to stay with my mother in Sherbrooke.

Several months after the accident, I returned to work. Emotionally I closed myself off from people and from myself. The guilt was too painful to face. On the outside I remained very sociable, but inside I erected a huge barrier to keep my guilt and emotions in check. This barrier prevented others from seeing my pain, and it stopped me from facing it. I was able to function normally, but just barely. I gave a tremendous amount of energy to my work and put a lot of other things on hold. I wasn't even aware of the people around me and the effect I had on them.

A little later, Lydia came to look for work as a teacher at the centre, and the two of us began a relationship. She was very caring and sympathetic. It was Lydia who helped me to move back to the house in St. Jean while Gavin stayed with my mother. When Gavin was almost two years old, he returned to live with me. In the evenings, after work, I rocked him, I played with him, but I was still in shock from the death of my wife. After Gavin's return, Lydia was at the house so often that she finally moved in, and we soon got married.

Lydia wanted to adopt Gavin. But there were delays, and I felt that he was my first wife's child. I somehow didn't want him to have another mother. Neither was I comfortable with the idea of having a second child. So, in the end, she didn't adopt him. But really, Lydia is the only mother Gavin knows.

Lydia was a very organized and capable woman. She provided Gavin and me with a certain routine. She gave our lives structure. She knew how to run a house. She had very precise ideas about how to live one's life, and this gave me a sense of security. She provided stability for both me and Gavin. But it couldn't last indefinitely. It's fine to be responsible, but when one of the two partners doesn't take responsibility, there is a tremendous weight on the other's shoulders. Now I can see that I didn't assume my rightful place in the relationship. I didn't assume my share of the emotional responsibility. I put her on a pedestal. I admired her. I thought that was love, but it wasn't. Far from it.

At the time I spoke very little. I was turned inward, preoccupied with myself. I could have a social conversation but I couldn't talk about emotions, about things that were meaningful. Lydia and I didn't have discussions. We communicated very little during our relationship. If the two of us went to a restaurant and she didn't talk, we didn't have much of a conversation. Not surprisingly, that began to bother her. In retrospect, I don't think I was very different from some of the mentally handicapped people I worked with at the centre.

As the years went on, I noticed that the physically and mentally handicapped children I worked with reached their maximum potential after a certain time and then diminished in capacity. This realization was very discouraging, but it forced me to reassess the meaning of progress. Perhaps what I had to give to these children was not about some cumulative result in the future. It had more to do with the quality of their lives in the present. So it became more important to me to try to reach them in the present than to teach them specific tasks.

To reach them and to teach them are very different things. Their way of communication is very different from our own traditional ways. The majority of the people I worked with didn't talk. What do you do when you spend eight hours alone with people who don't speak? You end up talking to them. You tell them what's going on, what you're doing, like the other teachers. But I began to wonder what my words meant to them. How did they interpret my words? How could they put my words to use? What would mentally handicapped people who cannot speak find stimulating? I had to become quite inventive in trying to reach them. And I became more sensitive in picking up and interpreting their reactions.

In time, I became better and better at devising new forms of communication. But the method of communication you develop with one is not necessarily adaptable to all handicapped. Each one is different. Some are not very sensitive to words and sound but are very sensitive to the sense of touch. Touching is a form of communication. So I took them to the woods, where they could touch trees, flowers, where they could have a physical communication with nature. And if touching does not provide the needed form of stimulation, you can always use affection. Slowly I began to wake up to the importance of communication, both during my work and outside.

⟨𝔰

Also, I learned to live with the unknown. I realized that you can't have expectations from the handicapped. You never know how they are going to act from one hour to the next. They challenge our definition of time. When you're with them, you have to learn to forget your own rhythm. You have to enter into their pace, their sense of time.

These days, because the disease has reached my throat and it takes me a while to get my words out, I often barely start a sentence and the person has left. People have little patience to wait for me to bring out what I want to say. Now I'm confronted by the average person in society, and I had spent eighteen years with people who had to face this same problem. Society has advanced considerably in its attitude toward the handicapped, but there's still a discomfort and an inability to try to understand another rhythm from one's own. Now it's my turn to have the experience from the other side. An interesting twist.

After working at the centre for several years, I began to get used to the handicapped, and because you're used to them you no longer think of them as handicapped. I began to discover fine and touching qualities about each one that were not at first discernible. As a result, my concept of beauty changed. Physically they didn't fit society's traditional definition of beauty, which only considers the facade. These young people were very deformed. You would think twice about kissing and hugging them. They don't obviously invite immediate physical affection. I needed to learn to give them affection. I needed to look beyond the surface for an internal beauty. But internal beauty is much more subtle. It takes time and sensitivity to find. It stretches your limits.

I was aware that the outside world was far from ready to accept these people or to give them a place. When I first took the handicapped youths for a walk in a shopping mall or a department store, I was immediately confronted by a lack of tolerance for differences. As I walked with these youths, people moved away from us. When someone dared to ask me a question about them, the first question was always, "Are these kids aggressive?" Certainly we did have a few who were aggressive, but look at what's happening in the world. Aggressiveness is not just for the mentally handicapped. People didn't even want to stay in a waiting room with an extremely handicapped person. In the dental clinic, the secretaries always put us ahead of the others to get rid of us as quickly as possible. People were very ill at ease. Their discomfort saved us from having to wait for hours, but you're also faced with a terrible lack of tolerance for anything different in society. I was daily forced to confront the meaning of normalcy.

My work taught me to question society's definition of normalcy. I began to think that perhaps there are numerous definitions of what's normal. You can't call a people normal just because they happen to be able to do certain things that are accepted by society. A lot of "normal" people need help and are incapable of dealing with areas that are not obviously perceptible. When I was with Lydia, I don't think I was functioning normally in my private life.

Lydia and I were married for twelve or thirteen years and tried to stay together for as long as possible. But divorce was inevitable. Luckily it was a very friendly divorce, partly because I think I was beginning to wake up and acknowledge my inability to be fully present in our marriage.

After the divorce, I found myself alone with Gavin. I had to organize our lives and take full responsibility. And I began to feel freer, as if something had loosened within. It was like the curtains had been drawn and the windows opened to allow light and fresh air to enter. I had more time for Gavin as well as more time for myself. And I had space to be alone. I actually discovered myself for the first time in my life. Before, I never even thought there was such a thing as "myself." Before, I had fled from myself. I hid from myself. Finally, I began to look at who I was.

❧

During my last five years at work, the centre opened a workshop geared toward weaning the students from the institution. We called this deinstitutionalizing them, helping them to eventually live in small groups, in houses. I was transferred to teach a group in the workshop. I was responsible for six people, all over twenty-one. Three were in wheelchairs and three were more mobile. The workshop did subcontracts for various companies. We had contracts to package screws. Each worker had to put a certain number of screws in individual bags. The most agile could close the bags.

I met Collette at the workshop. She contacted companies to obtain subcontract work for the handicapped. Soon after Lydia and I divorced, I found myself spending more and more time with Collette, having coffee or lunch in her office, talking to her after work. I found it easy to be with her. One day I suggested we see each other outside of work, and we quickly became good friends. I think I was open to such a relationship because I finally had time to be alone and think. I was becoming more open with myself, and Collette encouraged this openness. She was very dynamic. She talked easily and well, with a good vocabulary and a good command of language. She expressed her ideas very clearly. And she was at ease discussing her feelings and emotions. It was a pleasure talking to her, listening to her. Often, when I arrived home after spending the evening with her, I sat down to write a poem. Her willingness to be open inspired me. I wrote about objects, the weather, situations, other people. I wrote late in the evenings in the living room while Gavin was asleep. It was very quiet, peaceful. It was extraordinary.

Writing poetry gave me tremendous pleasure. It was the first time I did something for myself, for pure pleasure. And I had never before experienced such satisfaction. I allowed myself to be inspired, to be carried away by the pure joy, the pure delight of expression. Writing poetry was like a dream that had begun at CEGEP, when I wanted to be a writer. But as a student, I didn't have the capacity to express an inner passion. I was uncomfortable with my own emotions because they felt so unstructured. When we confront our passions, we can't always control ourselves. And when I was young, I was afraid of losing control. But this time, when I sat down to write, I allowed myself to face my passion, my emotions. Looking within and writing about what I found there became very important to me. I ceased to be afraid of my own feelings.

Collette and I easily spent two to three hours talking on the phone. We could spend four hours talking over dinner. There was no uncomfortable dead space between us, as I had experienced with Lydia. We talked about the difficulties of being open with oneself and others. We discussed our fears. Over time, our relationship became more and more intimate. Our conversations developed greater and greater depth. We talked about our desire to grow and the direction in which we wanted to grow. We talked about the conflicts that exist between people and why. We explored each other's psyche. All these discussions helped me to define myself. It was very exciting, stimulating. I felt myself very drawn to her.

I fell in love with Collette and wrote a poem which was a declaration of my love. I mailed it to her and asked her to send me a reply. I knew it would take two or three days for her to get my letter. One morning when I arrived at work, I immediately knew by the look on her face that she had received it. She looked quite disturbed. For two or three weeks we didn't speak to each other. I was willing to wait for her answer for as long as it took her to reach a decision. I was not going to pressure her in any way. At work she hardly looked at me. I knew I had taken a chance by telling her I loved her. I knew I could lose her as a friend. But I had to tell her. I had to do it for myself, to finally voice my feelings and take responsibility for the consequences.

One day she called me on the phone. She said she had always considered me a very good friend and didn't want anything more. And she didn't understand why I had fallen in love with her because she never flirted with me, never had any thoughts of going any further than friendship, and certainly never acted in any way seductive. I told her she didn't need to be flirtatious or seductive for me to have fallen in love with her. I simply fell in love with her as she was. But if friendship was all she wanted, we could continue as before. That would be enough for me. Though her reply was disappointing, I was very happy that I had proclaimed my feelings. For the first time in my life, I could tell a woman how I really felt.

It was a challenge for me to give expression to such a deep emotion. Early in my childhood, with my father's depression and drinking problem and the screaming matches between my parents, I was afraid to express my true feelings. To me, feelings were violent because my parents expressed themselves in such a violent way. Talking to Collette and writing poetry were surprisingly gentle and safe outlets for my emotions. They allowed me to gradually go deeper and deeper within myself till I discovered this love. To me, discovering and proclaiming this love were as important as concretizing it.

I kept all the poetry I wrote. Soon after the diagnosis Gavin said to me, "Why don't you publish some of the poems you've written, and after you go I'll have your book of poetry." I took him seriously. If he hadn't suggested that I publish my poems, I probably wouldn't have thought of it. But when I looked over what I had written to date, I found I didn't have enough for a book. And by then I had lost the use of my hands and could no longer write on my own. A number of friends offered to help. They told me to call them when I had composed a poem in my head, and they would write it down for me. As I got sicker, this was a way for me to continue writing poetry.

Publishing the book was the dream that kept me going. Dreaming is very important. It doesn't matter if the dream comes true or not. I dream of getting back my health. It's a wonderfully relaxing pastime.

By the time all the poems were finished, I was already in a wheelchair. I personally paid for the publishing of the book, and when it was done I had a launch. Over a hundred people showed up, and I gave each person a copy. Everything in there comes from my life, what I have lived and felt. Now I'm working on a second volume of poetry. Creating poems is an important source of expression for me. While composing words, thoughts, I forget my condition. I forget that I'm confined in a nursing home and live inside my head where there is infinite space. I am free.

CB

Before I worked with people in wheelchairs, people who depended on others. Now, I cannot move without a wheelchair, and I depend on others to do the most intimate things for me, just as others have depended on me. The situation I'm in brings back a lot of memories. At the workshop, I once had two women in wheelchairs under my care. When they had their menstruation, I was responsible for changing their sanitary napkins. It was part of my job. I felt comfortable doing it, but did I do it properly?

Now I know that being dependent on another for personal needs is very uncomfortable. Whether it's a man or a woman who takes care of my genital area, it's never the same as if I were to do it as an autonomous, independent person. Even with the best of intentions, it's impossible for another to take care of your personal hygiene the way you yourself would do it. Try to imagine that tomorrow morning another person will brush your teeth, wipe your behind, wash you. Think of how you touch yourself, soap yourself. You have your own way of doing it. No one can duplicate it. No matter how careful or caring someone is, no one can touch you the way you touch yourself while performing the most basic functions. The details I once took for granted I now become aware of because no one can duplicate them for me. It's incredible. If you're with someone who loves you and listens to you, and you're capable of giving them verbal directions, they'll do the best they can, but it's still not exactly the way you would do it for yourself. And imagine how tiring it is to give directions for every movement, especially for me who has difficulty talking. With the speed at which I talk, by the time I finish getting a bath, the water is cold.

If I could have my independence back and could take a bath or shower by myself, it wouldn't be like the routine it was before. I would take such pleasure in it. There is a pleasure and relaxation in being able to wash yourself that goes beyond the necessity of hygiene. I never thought about the value of such things before. I could have the most beautiful woman wash my body and it wouldn't be the same as doing it myself.

Usually women take care of my physical hygiene, and they aren't all comfortable with it. The first time a woman takes care of washing me, I feel I need to say something to make her feel comfortable, to add humour to a situation that could be uncomfortable for both of us. If a woman is comfortable, I feel much more relaxed and at ease. You would think that as a man I would enjoy being washed by different women. But I get no particular enjoyment out of it. I have absolutely no sexual reaction. The first time I was washed by a woman, I got an erection. It was like an automatic response from the past, I couldn't help it. She joked about it when she saw how uncomfortable I was.

No two women have the same touch. Some women have such a wonderful, pleasant touch that there is almost a chemistry between us. There are certain women who have a very sensual touch. It's an art for a person to take care of another person's physical hygiene. The way a person wipes you after you've been to the toilet, it's a whole art. But most of the time, when someone takes care of me, I feel like I'm being handled, like a dish being washed. Not that the people don't try their best, but inevitably they have to handle me with a certain efficiency, a certain routine. My body has become public. Physically, I simply have to forget that this is my body, it is no longer in my full possession to do with as I please. Physical intimacy just doesn't exist for me anymore. In spite of all this physical contact with others, I have no physical intimacy with myself, and at one point that created a real depression. The intimacy of my needs, like going to the bathroom, suddenly becomes part of a relationship, a social interaction.

When I'm moved from the wheelchair to a regular chair or from the wheelchair to the bed, that's a very close contact with another. Sometimes it's so close that I actually feel something quite strongly. When a person moves me from a wheelchair she has to bend down, take me under the arms, and, as she places me onto the chair or bed, she must bend down again, and they are totally unaware that their cleavage falls right at the level of my eyes and I can clearly see their breasts and bras. When that happens, it bothers me. I feel like my own sexuality doesn't matter anymore and no one takes account of it. They take so little account of it that they willingly expose themselves to me.

On a physical level, I still have all my sensibility intact, but I can no longer act. At one time I thought sexual intimacy meant genital contact. At a certain point in my illness that definition had to change. I have a friend with whom I have a very high level of intimacy that I would today call sexual. We've gone much farther than I would have thought possible. There is no sexuality in the traditional sense, but there is a depth of emotional exchange that I have never known before. There is a deep affection and tenderness. And we continue to evolve in our ability to be intimate, though we have never made love. For me, now, intimacy, sensuality, and emotional exchange go hand in hand.

This illness is helping me to explore avenues I never before realized existed. There is such a richness and depth of possibility to human communication, with the self and others. Through the poems people write down for me, I try to express the level of intensity that can exist in relationships. Before, I was afraid of intensity. Now, I seek it out. Before, I had problems expressing my feelings. Since my diagnosis, the emotional openness I've developed has helped to create a much stronger relationship with my son, and it has also brought me closer to my brothers and friends. Now, there is a greater depth to our discussions as well as our shared moments of silence.

In my condition, it would be easy to feel useless and without worth. But the feedback I get from family and friends provides me with tremendous emotional support and gives me a sense of my own value. They say they find me very courageous. Gavin has said he is proud of me because I write and because of the way I live my illness. Friends say I provide them with an example of how to be, that I've helped them in their personal search, a search that really doesn't have anything to do with me. They say I'm an inspiration to them. Through me they have learned to value and appreciate their own life.

CR

I, in turn, am exploring new ways to be. Since the diagnosis, I've embarked upon an internal journey which is not yet over. I'm searching for a state of serenity that will lead me toward a continuity, prepare me for the final departure. The effort to prepare myself is difficult and at the same time stimulating. Here in the nursing home, I've finally accepted my physical diminishment and everything that entails. Now, the final stage of the journey is spiritual. Perhaps there is no end to such a journey.

Every morning I pray. Prayer helps me to work toward serenity. Another good tool is my contact with other people. I might have an intimate conversation with the person who gives me a bath or feeds me, and we touch each other on a deep level. These are important moments for me. Everyone, including my brothers, my son, strangers, can be an agent sent to help me work on serenity. Being with others, feeling responsible for how I listen and what I say to them, all helps my work toward serenity. Time spent alone thinking is another important part of my daily life. In fact, it's absolutely necessary. Time alone is a little like a warm bath. It's relaxing and stimulating at the same time. So my three tools to work on serenity are prayer, the people around me, and time alone, silence.

When I was married to Lydia I also had spaces of silence, but it was a destructive silence. It's amazing how silence can be experienced in such a contradictory way. Now, I can live a silence of peace. I can pay attention to myself. The more time I spend consciously working on serenity, the larger my inner space seems to become. On the inner level, I continue to grow. There seems to be no limit. Just infinite space. My inner terrain is much larger than before, with a depth that continually amazes me. I now see that I must exercise certain aspects of myself to continue stretching this inner region. Silence is one form of exercise. For the first time in my life, I feel I'm taking an active role in my own evolution. I'm no longer a passive and helpless observer. But I'm finding that a by-product of this work on serenity is detachment. And sometimes that can be disturbing.

C3

I don't know what will happen when I die. But I do know that I'm not ready. When I think of dying, I'm afraid. I get nervous. When alone, I can start crying at the thought of dying. Everything I've told you is true, but the fear is also true. I'm afraid of dying because I don't want to leave the relationships I now have, though I know they will continue in spirit. I believe there is continuity after physical death. There is no loss. But having relationships of such depth is something new for me. It scares me to leave them. So I know I'm not yet ready for death.

If I can continue on the spiritual path I've begun, if I pay attention, I believe I will know when the time approaches for me to die. And then I will be prepared. And ready.

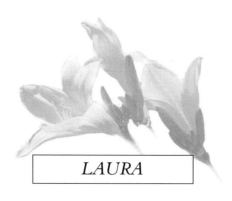

The same social worker who had given me Dianne's name also gave me Laura's name. She told me Laura, thirty-three and HIV positive, was seeing a therapist, and the social worker thought that talking to me would give her a good picture of her whole life. When I called her and stated my request, Laura replied in a voice full of energy and enthusiasm that she would be very interested in doing the interviews. We agreed to meet at her house.

She lived on the first floor of a small apartment building. Her one-bedroom apartment had a spacious, bright living room and dining room looking over a quiet, tree-lined street. Since all the interviews were at her home at ten in the morning, she met me at the door wearing a long, loose T-shirt with leggings, probably the clothes she had slept in. This changed over time to a bathrobe or just a loose T-shirt, but when we met in restaurants a couple of times for lunch or a coffee, she came very well dressed, in earth-tone designer clothes.

She had medium-length wavy blond hair, was small and finely built. The energetic voice belonged to someone quite grounded and practical. Her brilliant green four-foot lizard, called Tiger, comfortably sat across her chest during some of the interviews. Eventually, she also bought a little dog.

Throughout the interviews Laura was very open and straight-

forward, willingly answering all my questions. At times she was clearly
ashamed of some of the material she was relating. It is one thing to
talk to the girls in the dressing room of a strip club, bragging about
your ability to control a man, and quite another to talk to an outsider
in your pyjamas.

Laura related some of her stories with bravado, covering the pain
she must have felt at the time of the event. But occasionally — for
instance when she talked about her sado-masochism with her boy-
friend — she clearly felt uncomfortable: her voice dropped, her head
bent forward, and her eyes looked at the floor. She was viewing her
past with today's eyes and a changed perception.

As of this writing, in 2002, Laura's blood count is up to 400. She
is very much alive and active.

If I stop growing, if I stop doing what I'm doing right now, within six
months to a year I will die. I don't want the virus, but obviously I
must still need it. What I've learned to date hasn't been enough. I
don't know how much more I have to change, purify, and grow.

Over the last five years, my whole thinking and approach to life
got revamped. First, I had to learn to be open-minded, to stop being
stubborn, to stop rebelling. Rebellion has been a constant in my life,
against my parents, the system, the status quo. Even before getting
the virus, I was killing myself with my beliefs and attitudes. I lived
from crisis to crisis with a desperate confidence — "I know I'll make
it. I'll get through this."

As a junkie, you pull through a tough situation only to find the
next one is another jackpot. I thought I had screwed up so badly that
I had a real sense of unworthiness.

In AA people talked about a feeling of emptiness, a hole in the
gut. I was so far away from myself that I didn't even feel the hole. It
took a couple of years for me to get it. Before, I was always working
at making someone else happy so that I could finally be happy. Recently, I've had to become my own priority. And it's scary.

People in AA said, "You have to pass through the pain." I never understood that. Sometimes I would be fully sober and say, "I'm doing all the right things, how come I feel like a bag of shit?"

Now, when I have periods of emotional suffering, I know I'm going through something I need to learn this minute. And I know there is a very special gift waiting for me at the other end.

It's thanks to being sober long enough that I can see what I've been missing. I didn't realize life could be so gentle. I didn't realize people could have honest emotions. I just didn't think it was nice out here. Now I see so much beauty around me that I don't want to leave. It's crazy, isn't it?

Now I'm a strong believer that you use any help available. But my whole ability to reach out is new. Before, I didn't trust people. I just used them for my immediate needs, which was either money or drugs. Over the past year, Ann has become my healer, and Claire has become my psychologist. Ann helps me spiritually. Claire makes me look at things I don't want to see. She makes me review the past, helps me understand the pain. Before, I had no sense of chronology to my life. Everything was a jumble. She forced me to put my story together into a coherent whole. It took tremendous effort.

My first five years were spent in Glasgow, Scotland, with my grandparents. At the age of five, I found myself with these virtual strangers, my parents, who took me and a baby brother to Canada. My grandparents followed us a year later, and my grandfather died when I was eight. He was cremated, and his ashes were stored in my bedroom closet for three years. As a result, I was scared of the dark till I was twenty-nine and didn't dare tell anyone about it.

My parents came from impoverished backgrounds. In Canada, my father bought real estate, fixed up houses, and resold them. He was a man driven by goals. Now, he is a millionaire and still constantly working. I remember him as an authoritarian, a staunch Scotsman. No frills. Everything had to be functional, practical.

I always wanted to be a boy and was really into sports. I loved to go fishing with my dad. When my brother, who was two and a half years younger than me, was old enough to go, I was no longer invited. My father replaced me with his son, who didn't even like fishing. I was furious.

When I was around eight I was tested a lot because they wanted to send me to a school for exceptional children. That same year, my mother found out that both she and my brother were dyslexic. From then on, if my brother managed to pass, it was amazing and we had parties. If I got eighties everyone was disappointed. I constantly had to be working for A's. Anything other than perfection was not good enough.

Because my brother wasn't book smart, he tried to compensate by being the helpful son. Where I had a life, he enjoyed my parents' company. He sucked up to them. If I did anything my parents would frown upon, he would be the first to tell them about it.

I wasn't popular at school. I was prone to telling lies, which lost me a lot of respect, so I became a bully. I was small and got the biggest girls into the most trouble. Then they became my comrades, and I schemed with them. I had three girls, and we called ourselves the Bruisers. In grade seven, I started an extortion ring — "Pay up or we'll beat you up." Protection money. Lunch money. I was creating street gangs in upper-middle-class suburbia. I did it partly because I was low on the totem pole. Some kids were getting twenty dollars a week allowance. I was getting three dollars from my Dad and one dollar from my grandmother. I developed this tough-guy image as a survival tactic. Today, I'm five feet tall and one hundred and three pounds. I was probably even smaller then. My modus operandi has always been, the best defence is good offence. And it works.

I was terrible with authority figures. I didn't think they merited much respect. I was bright and caught things quickly. I thought they weren't as smart as me. My attitude was, challenge me and maybe then you'll get some respect. Until then, I'm running the school.

In seventh and eighth grade, I was also on a lot of barbiturates and amphetamines. My girlfriend's mother was a total basket case who had monster bottles of pills in her medicine cabinet. She didn't notice if twenty were gone. I was on a roller coaster for two years.

⚘

The beatings began as I started getting into trouble. Every time I got hit, I went out and did something else. Soon my father was beating me regularly. The last three years I lived at home, I constantly had a bruise on my body. The only time my mother ever intervened was when my father broke my nose.

What I got from my father, I gave to my brother. I remember absolutely hating him because he had a lot of goods on me. He threatened to tell my parents that I was having sex with my boyfriend. When I was about twelve or thirteen, I hated him so much I raped him. I pinned him down, got on top of him, and put his cock in me. I said, "Now tell them I'm having sex." After that, he just clammed up. I felt that if I had that on him, he couldn't use any of the cards he had up his sleeve.

For years, I didn't even remember what I had done. When I was eighteen, after a bad LSD trip, the memory came flooding back. It was so vivid, the smells, the sounds, the feeling of power I had the day I did it. I felt just horrible about it. As I was getting sober this was a real issue. In AA they say, "Make amends to all people wherever possible, except when to do so would injure them or others." I pussyfooted around the issue in a couple of letters I sent him.

By the time I was thirteen, I was getting into trouble with the police, which increased the beatings. Children's Aid ordered us to see a psychologist. I went with my parents. My father was asked to stop hitting me to see if I was really wayward or if I was acting out because of the beatings. He got really pissed off. He said he had been raised like that and nothing was wrong with him. We never went back.

By then, I was already experimenting with leaving home. One weekend we took a girlfriend's father's truck for a joyride, and it ran out of gas on the highway. Everyone started panicking and took off. They left me with this enormous one-and-a-half-ton truck. Somehow I had to get it back. I knew how to drive it, I had learned on other cars we had taken for joy rides. I just needed gas. I walked to the next exit, to a phone, and called a girlfriend, who put me on to Wesley, her thirty-eight-year-old boyfriend. He offered to come down and tow me to a gas station.

By the time we got the truck back, it was already one in the morning. I crashed it backing into the parking spot, but at least it was there. I couldn't go home at that hour. Wesley offered to put me up in a hotel room. He made it really easy for me not to go home. Two weeks later, he made a move and I felt I owed him something.

Then the police found me and took me back home. My dad said, "Take her somewhere to be disciplined."

They said, "She just ran away. We can't put her in a detention home."

I went to my room. After the police left, my father called me out. That was the second time I saw him cry. He said, "You know we love you."

I was so angry with him I said, "That's too fucking little, too fucking late." I went back to my bedroom and climbed out the window.

I ran back to Wesley. At the time he was making fifteen hundred or two thousand dollars a day doing fraud, and he spoiled me. Wesley was a rather ugly man, not physically appealing in the least. It was his money I liked. He took me shopping. I was eating at McDonald's all the time. For a thirteen-year-old, that's spoiled, especially in my family, where we never went to a restaurant. I could stay up till all hours of the night. When we moved into an apartment together, he bought me a German shepherd named Zeus. And I was like his wife. I did his laundry. I cooked and cleaned.

I was with him for no more than two months when I found out he had two sons from a previous relationship. They were four and six when I met them. Then I became mother to the kids.

The first two years, I was the perfect little housekeeper. I cut radishes into little flowers for supper, bought only the products advertised on TV. I was meticulous about everything.

By the time I was fourteen, I held three jobs. I was geared for success. During the day I did telephone soliciting and got promoted to receptionist. At night, I worked for a disco as a coat check girl and for a taxi company as a midnight dispatcher.

Then Wesley got busted for fraud. A few days later, he got out of jail, and we moved in with his parents. Wesley's father was a pedophile who had just gotten out of Kingston Penitentiary for having murdered a twelve-year-old boy he had buggered. He had done his time.

Later, Wesley and I bought three acres of land in the country and constructed our own house. He put up six-foot fences with barbed wire at the top and flood lights all around. He said, "I want to see them coming."

He lived in constant fear and paranoia.

That same summer, he started an excavation company, and I saw him take a body bag from the trunk of the car and bury it with the bulldozer. I was scared. Also, there were always guns around. Later, I found out he was a contract killer for the mob.

By the time I'm fifteen I end up pregnant. From that point on, everything changed because I wasn't a little girl anymore. Wesley began beating me. But I loved being pregnant, especially when I got very big and he used to go away for days and days at a time. I used to talk to Chad. I had named him before he was even born. I was setting the baby up to go to his new mom, Carol, a friend of mine. It was all arranged. I was going to be known as the aunt and was never going to lose contact with him.

I didn't really want to give him up. After he was born, while I was still in the hospital, I had a dream. When I wanted to give him up in my dream, the nurses and doctors chased me. I ran with Chad in my arms and tripped. The baby flew into Carol's arms, and she turned around, all white, and said, "He's dead."

When he was three months old, he died. Crib death. And I blamed myself.

After Chad died, I went to see my parents in a $300 business suit, $150 Gucci shoes, and a short mink jacket. By then they had bought a farm. As my father was showing me around, he said I could come back. He said he understood that I had been through some things that wouldn't allow me to move back into the house, and I should pick a piece of land on which he would build me a small bungalow.

We hiked around the property, and I found the spot I wanted. When we came back to the house, Dad ran upstairs to wash up, and Mom and I were sitting in the kitchen. She said, "I hope you're not planning to move back."

I said, "What do you mean?"

She said, "I'm not going through the same troubles I had with you the first time."

"You know what, Mom, the thought never crossed my mind."

After that, I went back to Wesley, did check fraud, and began to drink.

Wesley's female friends were all prostitutes. These girls had money and nice clothes. They had everything a sixteen-year-old in a depression could want. One of them was a call girl who was absolutely beautiful, very classy. That's the girl I modelled myself after. She explained how to do it. Then I got into prostitution. Wesley didn't mind. It always boiled down to dollars and cents.

At this time we were living with Wesley's parents again. I was like a slave. I was helping out with the bills through prostitution. I was cleaning house. I was taking care of the kids.

For quite a while, I had been trying to leave Wesley. I just kept getting caught at it. Either I would be pinched when I was packing my bags, or I would be storming out of the house and he'd follow me in the car. One day his father said, "You want out? Pack your bag now. I'm taking you."

By helping me get away, he was giving it to his son, whom he really didn't like.

Wesley managed to find me because I was still working out of the same hotels. He got hold of my book of clients and called each one to tell them I had the dose. I offered him money to get him off my back. We agreed to meet at a restaurant. I paid the biggest, blackest guy I could find to come with me. Everything was prearranged. At the restaurant, I provoked Wesley to get really angry, and when he raised his hand to hit me, this black guy dragged him outside and kicked the shit out of him. He never bothered me again.

By the time I was seventeen, I was doing crystal Methedrine, bathtub speed. In the late 1970s bikers all over the world were making it up in bathtubs. A year later, I met this guy as a client who put me up in a suite at the Holiday Inn. I was living in fine style and wasn't paying for anything. Then it started clicking that this wasn't going to be as easy as it appeared. At that point, I called up my dad and asked one of the single most stupidest questions ever. "What's the Mafia?"

He explained that they were drug dealers and smugglers who lived off the avails of prostitution. I went, "Oh, can I come home?"

He said, "You've been gone for five years. I don't think you can come back."

A couple of months later, I moved into my own apartment but still continued to see this guy. One night, he saw me do a line of coke and slapped me across the face. At this point, I was paying for the apartment from prostitution. I had bought him a gold watch. I was giving him money. When he slapped me, it was like, you're yesterday's news. I don't need you.

Then I got arrested for check fraud. I got three years probation and decided to get out of town. In Montreal, I became a street whore. Everything was done at lightning speed. I prided myself on being down, up, and cash in my hand in ten minutes. That's undressing, washing, everything. Done. Ten minutes. The girls used to be amazed. We had races. That's how we made the job interesting.

I've never had any bad experiences with tricks. In that capacity, I can be totally honest. I can say what I'm going to do and do what I say. Also, I'll take the time to listen to someone. A lot of people are starved emotionally. It made me feel good to be there for them. I felt I was doing a service. I used to have this trick who ended up dying of multiple sclerosis. None of the other prostitutes would see him because he was physically twisted. But he was the nicest guy in the world, and he was one of my favourite customers because he appreciated me so much.

CB

Then I got into the bar scene and started stripping. By the time I was twenty, I met Gary. He was a trick who gave me way more money than most. A lot of money is always a hook for me. I think, If he's got that much money, it must be secure. At that point I was physically tired. Mentally worn out. I had reached bottom with the drugs and prostitution. Gary, who was twelve years older than me, was a way out.

We moved to California together because he wanted to get out of the mob. He taught me how to grow marijuana in the mountains. And he took an interest in me. He listened to what I had to say. He told me I was bright. He was very much in love with me. After two and a half years in California, the mob found him, and he was asked to come back to Montreal.

Once back, I helped Gary with drug smuggling. Chinese heroin coming from Amsterdam to Montreal. A guy in Holland made boxes with false bottoms and false sides for us. Inside the boxes were Delft vases. I picked up the packages at the airport and paid taxes on the vases. After a while, the vases became suspicious. Then we got into crating animals: snakes, alligators, and big dogs. Customs officials didn't particularly want to look inside a box marked: attention live reptile.

I started stripping again, but this time with a difference. Stripping as a career started with Gary. Because he was a promoter and an agent for bands, he had a sense of showmanship. I had been a competitive gymnast as a child, and no one had ever said, "You can put a cartwheel in your act."

He did. He taught me glitz. Suddenly I acquired the sequins, the feather boas, the three-quarter-length gloves, the garter belt, the hose, the hairdos, and the nails. Flashy, trashy, that's my gig. When costumes entered my world, I was a star. With Gary's help, I became a performer as opposed to just a dancer. I did my sets to classical or blues music. You didn't hear that in the clubs. Where did Vivaldi come in? Who's on stage? Customers loved it.

Gary and I used to have breakfast at the same café every morning.

One of the waiters was a choreographer who had a dance troupe. He owed Gary some money for grass. One day Gary said, "Jacques will pay me by giving you dance lessons."

Perfect, a private choreographer. We went to his loft, and he asked me why I wanted the dance lessons. I said, "I'm a stripper, and I'd like to improve my show. I want to fly through the air."

He said, "We'll start with the basics."

With Jacques, I learned to slow down. Before, I had been driven by movement. As a gymnast, I had been taught to hit the target, make the flip, land on two feet. I didn't think about aesthetics. Jacques taught me grace and fluidity.

Then Gary started talking about settling down. He had already done everything I still wanted to do. I wanted more adventure, excitement. When I left him, I started hitting the skids, doing a lot more drugs and booze. I stayed awake for three to five days straight, using coke. Then I crashed for a day or two. Then it started all over again. I did that for about a year and a half before I met Tom.

I was still in touch with Gary, who had bought a blues club. I went over one night and saw this striking, six-foot-four blond guy with green eyes. An incredible figure of a man. It was lust at first sight. I asked him if he had anything to smoke. He said, "I've got some grass back at my apartment."

When we got there, he said, "I don't have any grass, but I have coke." He pulled out a needle, and when he did his hit, I saw him register. I saw him get the immediate effect of the drug. I just took his needle and made myself a hit. We ended up having sex and drugging the whole night. I was to be on the needle for five years after that.

I knew from the moment it started I shouldn't be in it. He was very aggressive. I saw him stealing from people. I saw him doing crooked deals. Where I was from, drug dealers were gangsters with ethics. He was a punk. I thought, You've got to get away from this guy. And I couldn't. I stayed for the drugs. And the whole showmanship of my work went out the window.

He became my doctor. He shot me up, and I got lost in the needle. Because he was my doctor, I don't have the kind of track marks most people do who shoot themselves up. You see people with abscesses, holes in their hands, holes in their jugular, and they're bruised. If it's done properly, there's no bruising, no abscessing. There is a whole aesthetic to marks.

I moved in with him. Every cent I made went into drugs. I started prostituting again. I was making money hand to mouth. We were living in tourist rooms. Then we moved in with a man who was a terrible alcoholic and needed someone to cook his meals and clean house. It was a rent-free place to use our drugs. That got me back on my feet where I could work again.

Six months after we had been together, Tom went for a bioresearch study and his blood test came back positive for HIV. Since we had been sharing needles, he suggested I be tested. My results also came back HIV positive. My blood count was 370 at the time of diagnosis. I asked how much longer I had to live. They said the average was about eighteen months. I was sure they were right. Okay, I'm going to party till it's over. I kept drugging and drinking for the first eighteen months.

Soon after he was diagnosed, Tom decided to go back to finish high school. That year, I didn't have money to buy him a birthday gift and offered to do his paper for a sociology course. At the time, he was always calling me stupid. He got an 86 on the paper I wrote, and I realized I wasn't as stupid as he said. From then on, I did all his term papers, and he always got good marks. I thought, If I can do it for him, I could do it for me. I decided to go back to finish high school myself.

Tom told me I was wasting my time. I put the alarm clock on, and he turned it off. He definitely didn't like me going back to school. For the first couple of semesters, I was consistently on the honour roll. Then the junk got too bad. I was shooting up at school, was caught, and got kicked out.

After a while, we moved out of this guy's apartment into another one in the same building. By then, I was getting regular beatings. I was with that man for five years, and there wasn't a day that I didn't have a bruise. Just like living with Dad. Tom didn't work. I was supporting him, but that didn't stop him from beating me. He beat me so badly that I was in hospital four times. Three times, when I was beaten unconscious, the ambulance had to come and get me. Tom went to jail five times for beating me up because a neighbour had called the police. Every time he was in jail, I ended up working regularly and buying something new for the house.

After eighteen months, I woke up one morning and realized I wasn't dead. That's when my thinking started to change. By then, I knew I was really strung out. The needle had brought me to my knees. I knew I first had to change that behaviour before I could change anything else. But I still loved my drug. I still loved my needle. I loved the notoriety, the whole look, dressing in black, being a rebel. I loved the fact that I was living a style others wouldn't dare attempt. In my mind, everybody wanted to be doing what I was doing. To risk. Every time I put a needle in my arm, I was risking my life. And everyone wants to be a risk taker. My track marks were like a badge of courage, a badge of daring. And it was important that I survive well. I could do my dope and still have my place. I knew other junkies who were living on the street as prostitutes. They'd turn a trick, do coke, turn another trick, more coke. I didn't work like that. I bought in quantities with money I made from stripping and prostitution. Or stealing. Whatever it took. I always made sure I had money. Nobody pulled off this junkie stunt quite as well as I did. Except those who were born wealthy.

Tom had introduced me to the needle, and I had introduced him to bondage and discipline. The first time we had sex together, it was bondage and discipline, something I had been experimenting with on and off throughout the years, with clients, with lovers. The bondage and discipline escalated and became S&M.

Tom began to dress up as a woman, that's how he wanted to be dominated. At first he put on my lingerie, which stretched. Then he sent me out to buy special underwear for him. I did his makeup. And I beat him as a woman. At first, the cross-dressing with Tom was an adventure because it was really stretching the limits of convention.

But the more we got involved in S&M, the bigger that part of him became. After the second year there was no sex at all, just S&M.

The S&M and the drugs were totally linked. Before I got ready to do the drugs, I was also preparing the stage for whatever was going to happen that night. I'd be pulling out gadgets from the drawer, or I'd think about what I was going to wear. Before doing the S&M, we shot up. I never stuck a needle in my arm unless I already had eight ounces of booze in me, and I never did S&M unless I was already high on coke. During S&M, it wasn't uncommon for me to shoot up every fifteen minutes. I used to wear my watch so I could time when I'd be getting my next hit. After a while, the S&M got to be very repetitive. I got so sick of it one time that I hired a prostitute to do it for me.

S&M progresses. It gets more and more dangerous, more and more degrading. Even as a mistress, I passed boundaries I didn't think I would. Tom asked me to urinate on him. Then he'd beat me up the next morning — Look what you made me do!

I did nipple piercings on him. We went past the line where most people would stop. I saw a TV show once where someone was murdered during an S&M trip, and it really spoke to me.

There is an excitement element in how far you can push your body before it becomes too painful, and that's part of the gratification. It's a way to feel. S&M is where love and hate meet. Pleasure and pain. Only recently did I learn that something doesn't have to be threatening to be exciting.

There were times when I was actually longing to have a different kind of sex. Even straight sex would have been fine. One night, I was so fed up with what we were doing that I said, "For once, can't we just go out for dinner and score some drugs. Something normal." Also, I felt he was always the focus, and I would have liked the focus to shift to me sometimes. This cross-dressing can be very self-centred.

Once I ran away from Tom and did a six-day run. I was shooting up the whole time, didn't sleep, didn't eat. I was taking Boost, a supplementary diet drink. Then I went to the club and danced for a guy who was the son of a Guatemalan diplomat. He said to me, "Why are you starving yourself? You're so beautiful."

At that point, I hadn't eaten in five days. What he said hit home. This guy was from a country where people actually do starve to death.

From time to time I would be out on a run and scared to go back home because I was sure to catch a beating. I began to show up in women's shelters. After a couple of days, I started being able to eat again, and I called Tom to say, "Listen, this is what happened, I didn't mean to go out and use for three days, but I did. I'll come back if you promise not to hit me." Sometimes that worked, sometimes it didn't.

The women at the shelter treated me with respect, and I hadn't had that in years. They fed me. They gave me clothes, bus tickets. They were nice for no reason. At the time I was so into the junkie mentality that I really thought I was pulling one over on them. "Hah, I get a free place to stay and free meals."

The women's shelters put me in touch with Alcoholics Anonymous and Narcotics Anonymous. They also sent me to a detox centre because I was obviously a junkie. In detox, they realized they weren't going to lure me in with the prospect of good health. They lured me in with the prospect of free clothes, free meals, and a chance to get away. "Look upon it as a vacation," they said. And it worked for me. Tom had been through detoxes and rehabs himself. He knew what it was.

I stayed at the detox centre for six weeks. Six weeks without drugs or alcohol. The first seven days, you can't leave the facility, and slowly they give you privileges and bus tickets. I spent my days in the parks and my nights at AA meetings. The detox had suggested I go to the meetings. But I was doing everything for approval. I was going to be the best little detoxer. I didn't realize I had a life-threatening illness. For me everything was a game. I did two six-week detoxes before I realized, Oh, they're trying to tell me I have a problem with drugs and alcohol.

At first I didn't really know why I was at AA. I had no idea what they were talking about. I refused to stay for the Lord's Prayer because I had to hold hands with people, and I thought that was horrid. Also, I didn't know if I believed the words. It says, "Forgive us our trespasses as we forgive those who have trespassed against us, and lead us out of temptation." I didn't know if I wanted to be led out of temptation or if I wanted to forgive those who had wronged me.

When they told me, "You can rely on a power higher than yourself," I thought, "Perfect, if anybody can understand me it would be Him, if anyone can forgive me it would be Him." I was ready to believe in God.

When people first come into AA, they rely heavily on the support of other alcoholics. Not me. In the beginning, I wasn't even willing to tell people my story because I didn't trust anyone. God was the only thing I could buy into. Spirituality was the only thing I saw lacking in my life. Also, I quickly found comfort in the Serenity Prayer. "Thy will, not my will be done." I said that as a mantra before I even knew what a mantra was.

A month before I came into recovery, things began to happen. While out on a run, I would black out after two or three drinks and come to with a needle in my arm, on a hit, and I didn't know how much I had put into the syringe. At home, with Tom, I overdosed four times. I had had overdoses before but never so clustered. The more you overdose, the longer it takes to come back, and the more likely you are to die. By the end of the month, I was getting scared. I knew I had to leave Tom because the beatings were getting much worse. I knew I wouldn't have the strength to leave while still using.

One day, I got home from a six-day run, totally wrecked. Three days later, Tom wouldn't let me out of the house. He held me hostage. I knew I had to devise some plan to get out of there. I explained that I was sick with a drug and alcohol problem and needed to go to an AA meeting. He agreed to let me go. Often, he came to check up on me to make sure I was where I said I was. At times, he actually dragged me out because I had been gone too long. I stayed sober for a week, and Tom agreed to let me go back to work. I then opened a bank account and put half of everything I made in there, unbeknown to him.

Six weeks later, he was making burgers for dinner. He always cooked. I set the table, put out the condiments, and got ready for work. He sat down and noticed I had forgotten to put out the mustard. He took the huge, solid-oak dining room table and threw it across the room. Then he gave me the beating of my life because there was no mustard on the table. It was summer, I ran out of the house in bare feet because I didn't have time to put on shoes. I ran to a phone booth, called a girl I had met at AA, and told her what had happened. She said, "Come here right now." I went over to her house. Two weeks later, I asked the police to come back with me to pick up my clothes. Nobody from AA wanted to help me move out. They were scared of Tom.

When I left Tom, I was six weeks sober. I hadn't used the needle for six weeks. I only had to sober up for that long to be able to leave him.

The police escorted me back to the apartment. These cops had been there several times before for him beating me, when Tom came out, looking so dejected and perplexed, and said, "Why are you doing this? I've never done anything to you. We can work this out."

One cop said, "Sit down and shut up."

I packed six green garbage bags, which represented my worldly accumulation up to that point. I called a taxi. By the time I got into the cab with my garbage bags, I was crying because I was leaving my dog behind and I loved her.

En route, the taxi driver started telling me a story about a guy with no legs who was the happiest man in the world. And I felt so much better. It was crazy. My life as I knew it was over, and this taxi driver is telling me about this guy with no legs. I thought, Well, if he can be happy with no legs and has to go through life on a little wooden board with wheels, compared to him I have everything going for me.

Tom started hanging out at AA meetings to talk to me. He said he understood that I had to leave but he didn't have groceries and the dog was sick. I gave him a hundred dollars a week and paid the vet bills. Four months later, I had a relapse, and I just couldn't continue. Then he faded out of the picture.

I managed to stay sober for another four months. Then I met Michael in AA, only to get hooked on heroin with him. But at least I was conscious of what I was doing. I knew heroin was wrong.

Michael showed me the other side of midnight. Not only was he incredibly good-looking and absolutely charming, he owned his own business, he owned cars, had his own house. I was really impoverished when I was on the needle. I never saw things in terms of what money could do other than buy drugs. This guy dazzled me.

Then I set him up. I told him I had been tested for HIV and probably was positive because one of my girlfriends was dying with it, and we should practice safe sex. Three weeks later, I told him I had tested positive, pretending I had just found out. Then he wasn't sure about the relationship for six months, even though we still stayed together. During those six months, I took care of Michael. I made sure he was eating properly, sleeping properly, getting to work on time. I listened to him. I made myself indispensable.

When we started getting serious, I moved in with him. Then he wanted the perfect Jewish housewife. I'm not Jewish, but I'm teachable. He gave me books on Judaism. I started keeping a kosher kitchen. I became the good Jewish housewife, which offered me an identity.

For fourteen months, I didn't go to AA. During that time, I learned about neighbours, keeping house, mowing the lawn, taxes, earning a real salary. And I learned about running a business. Michael didn't want me to continue working as a stripper and said, "Come into the sheet metal business, and we'll make it a family affair." He had inherited the company from his father, who had just died. I went in and loved it. I was in my element, a natural.

Here I was doing the books, keeping ledgers, taking them to an accountant. I scheduled appointments. Did payroll. It came easy to me. But Michael wasn't committed to the business. He could deposit money but just couldn't leave it there. His partner also was after a lot of money. Within six months, they were so in the red they were panicking. I said, "Don't touch the money. Let me handle it."

After two months, I bought them a new truck. Then Michael took over the books again. We lasted through the winter, but I had to go back to stripping to support the company.

I was working hard, putting all my money from stripping into the business to keep it afloat, but I wasn't getting any respect for the contribution I was making. Michael was putting me down for being a stripper, but he still took my money. By June I had a relapse.

A little later we bought a four-bedroom bungalow in the suburbs, and I decided that I was going to renovate the house. Instead of putting all my money into the business, I'm now putting it into the house. I stayed sober for six months. Once the house was finished, I again started putting money into the business. I wanted it to survive. I was just starting this new way of life. I needed to be needed. I needed the status of living in the suburbs. I had arrived from needles to a bungalow with a garage and yard. I wanted to hold onto that.

Michael just wasn't that interested in the business. Then he had an affair. I found out about it and ended up getting drunk again and using cocaine. I had thought that if you could stay sober for six months, you could stay sober for six years, for good. The relapse scared me. I went to a treatment centre. After I got out, I decided not to put another dime into the business. I had to let it go. Six weeks later, it closed.

Then I got pregnant. At first I considered keeping the baby. I thought, "I have the kid, I tax myself, I die. Or if I don't die, the kid is born positive and dies in two and a half years." The risk of having another baby die weighed heavy on me. Or he doesn't get the disease, everything goes well for me, but he's seven years old, and I die. I knew

Michael was irresponsible. He wouldn't take care of the baby. Time was passing. The abortion finally won out.

I didn't have money for the abortion. Michael was in treatment at the time, and that was costing money. I needed money for heating oil. I was paying for everything. One day I went to the hospital to see my doctor, and in the hall Claire, the psychologist, came up to me and said, "Listen, I know of you. If there is anything you ever need, call me."

I called her and said, "Is there any agency that can help me out?"

She said, "Sure," and came up with a check the same day.

Then Michael decided he was going to sell the house. I didn't want him to sell it. I had put a lot of time, money, and love into that house. He didn't listen. When the sale was finalized, I relapsed again. Once more I was living on Boost. I wasn't eating, I wasn't sleeping. I realized that no one was going to take care of me except me. When I got sober again, I went back to finish high school. Then I took a computer course because I wanted to get a real estate license. Michael didn't like me going to school. He would say, "Baby, please don't go. Let's go shopping." He kept me up to all hours of the morning. He made it hard for me.

One Thanksgiving, I made a huge supper and invited ten people. I told them if they found anyone without a turkey to eat to bring them along. Eighteen people showed up. One of the women who came said she was a healer. I had met her at AA meetings and wouldn't trust her with my health. But I was interested in what she had to say about energy, chakra balancing, and meditation. I explained I had HIV and asked her if she could recommend someone. She said, "I have a girlfriend, Ann, who works with exceptional cancer patients." I got the number.

By then someone in AA had lent me a few meditation tapes. I had started practicing meditation. I was reading Louise Hay, M.F. Fox. By then I knew something had to change.

I called Ann and made an appointment. The first time I saw her, she said, "Oh, you have HIV, you have not been living your will. Somebody or something has been imposing its will on you. If it's a man, get rid of him."

"Sure, you make it sound so easy."

Soon after that, my blood count went down by 100, to 180. Instead of being just HIV positive, I was now considered to have full-blown AIDS. The day my doctor told me my T-cells had dropped, I saw Claire again in the hospital, and she said, "Is there anything I can do for you?" I knew I needed help and decided to start seeing her on a regular basis.

The news of having full-blown AIDS sent me into a depression. I quit all my courses and dropped out. I lived on Boost again. Never in my wildest imagination did I think my T-cells would go below 200. At that point Michael went out and drank again, after having been sober for four months. He thought he had the perfect excuse. Oh, my girlfriend is dying. I thought, "You piece of shit. First of all, I'm not dying. Second of all, you should be helping me, I shouldn't have to help you."

Then he got arrested for disturbing the peace while drunk. When he was in jail, I convinced him to go to a treatment centre, and I split. That was hard. Michael was a terrible thing to cut from my life.

Seeing Ann on a regular basis gave me the courage to leave him and move out on my own. I grew up a lot when that happened. I took responsibility. For the first time, I began to pay attention to myself. For Michael I could pay bills, for myself it didn't really matter. I can nurture others, but I don't count. It was even hard for me to feed myself. Ann counselled me on nutrition, vitamin supplements, and meditation. Now I like to cook. I can usually tell how healthy I am by how much cooking I'm doing.

I didn't leave Michael because I didn't love him anymore. I left because he was so unhealthy for me. Then that space gets filled up with David, who is so healthy and who is probably one of the nicest men I have ever known in my whole life. And at this point I'm healthy enough to allow that to happen.

Since David has arrived in my life, I've been very angry with my disease. I've been writing it letters, saying, "I really hate having you here." But there have been other times when I've written letters of gratitude. "Thank you for coming into my life to open my eyes. Thank you for allowing me to learn how to trust." This HIV hasn't been all bad.

Sometimes when I meet pitfalls in my recovery, I end up reverting back to old behaviour. One of the big signs that I'm in trouble is if I'm arranging to go and see a client for sex. It's an old behaviour. Approval seeking, controlling through sex, need to have money, need to have power.

Most people who follow the twelve-step program in AA find that the first step is just an unburdening. The second and the third is when the spiritual benefits come. I was four months sober when I did my first fourth step in AA, which is about resentment, fear, and sexual misconduct. I realized my first major block was resentment. I took my resentments one at a time. The three big ones were Wesley, my father, and Michael. As soon as I allowed myself to forgive these people, which took tremendous work, I felt almost immediate results. I felt physically lighter, stronger. As soon as the people who had hurt me were out of my head, it gave me room to think about myself, and I was able to eat properly, sleep properly, hire healers, go to therapists, go back to school.

Tom was the first person I forgave. He had gone through the same rehab as I had, and at one of the reunions he came over and asked me if we could talk. We went outside, and I could see he was upset. I said, "What's going on?"

His eyes filled with tears.

I said, "My God, what happened?"

The night before he had been shooting up with his new girlfriend, and I'm sure he had given her the hit because he had always given me mine. Her heart had exploded, and she died. That was as heavy as Tom had ever seen. For the first time, I saw him as an object of pity. What he was inflicting upon himself was much worse than what I could have wished for him.

After you work on your resentments, then you work on your fears. It took me three tries before I finally got results. When I started to face my fears, I didn't like it. I didn't want to do this. But so much healing had taken place when I released my resentments that I thought, Okay, it's fear now. I could see that I was afraid to be alone, I was afraid that I was going to die, I was afraid that I would lose certain friends, I was afraid there wasn't going to be any money. As soon as I put my fear of the dark into words, as soon as I told somebody, I could see it, and there was nothing to be scared of. In looking at fear, I saw how I acted, and I became more aware. I could catch myself. I'm always setting up scenarios to manipulate a situation so that it will work for me. But I'm always afraid of what the consequences will be if I get caught. As the fears came up, I faced them, and every time I faced them it got a little easier. Then I went on the hunt for fears. I was going around for months saying, "Yes, I love facing my fears, I go looking for fears so that I can conquer them."

When I got into the sixth step, "You are entirely ready to have God remove all these defects of character," I was immediately confronted with myself. I had to be willing to let go of my usual way of operating in life. Otherwise, I could see I was destined to repeat the same pattern. I saw a lot of situations where I was being manipulative, dishonest, irresponsible. I had to work through all of them, and it became just an amazing effort. I had to keep going over each defect again and again till I could clearly see the impact it had on my life and was finally ready to release it.

Because of the effort I devoted and continue to devote to my spiritual and physical healing, my blood count went up 100 points. Today, I'm not full blown-AIDS. And I might be able to heal myself of this HIV. I'm trying to do everything that's suggested to me. Some things fit better into my life than others, and those stay, like prayer and meditation. I'm also practicing the word no. I used to always bend myself out of shape to help someone else out, especially a man, to put his priorities first. Now I'm trying to put myself first. That's why I live alone today.

CS

I judge my inner balance on how well I meditate and how much I'm getting out of my meditation. Now I can feel what my needs are, and I look for specific meditations to fulfill them. Before, I didn't even know what my needs were.

Working with Claire on a regular basis helped me realize I wanted to reconnect with my parents. And that was one of the hardest things I've ever done. I went back very humbled, feeling that I had been a great disappointment. At first, establishing a fresh relationship with them was very painful, but over the last four years, my mother and I have become the best of friends, partly because she was so prepared to take responsibility for what had happened when I was a kid. Two Christmases ago, she told me that when I was eight, after she had been diagnosed dyslexic, she had cut me off emotionally because she was afraid I would find out she was stupid. She consciously decided not to talk to me more than necessary. She saw me as getting too far ahead of her. When she told me that, it put a lot of pieces into place. I was very thankful she admitted it. We had never before shared that level of honesty.

When I came back four years ago, my brother refused to see me or talk to me. At the time I was just starting AA, and I sent him a letter. I explained that I was sorry for my estrangement from the family, it was because I was an alcoholic and hoped that he could forgive me and now I was ready to reestablish ties. Would he consider seeing me or talking to me over the telephone? I got no response. He said to my mother, "I won't talk to her until I see that she's putting in a reasonable effort to be a part of this family." Now, I've done that, including remembering to send birthday cards.

A year and a half ago, I said to my mother, "I really feel that I've been toeing the line. Please, talk to Giles and tell him I want to see him."

She said, "He won't talk to you ever again, Laura."

I said, "Why not?"

Then she asked, "Did you once say that your father was sexually molesting you?" I didn't remember this episode at all. But tears immediately sprang to my eyes when she asked, and I knew it was true. I started crying and said, "I don't know. I really don't know."

Much later, I went back to my mother and said, "It's true. I did say that." When I was twelve years old, I had started a rumour that my father was sexually molesting me. The rumour must have gotten back to my brother. In reality, I was getting regular beatings, but that wasn't something I could complain about. In my family, getting a beating was normal.

This New Year's, I finally told my parents I had HIV. I expected my father to be a pillar of strength and my mother to fall apart. Instead, my father fell apart and my mother was the pillar of strength. Unfortunately, it threw a wrench into the relationship between my father and me. He's certain I'm going to die.

Before I told my mother about the HIV, she was just a friend. Before, she knew I had to be the strong, independent daughter I had always been. As soon as I allowed her to see my weakness, I allowed her to be a mother. Then she could show concern and ask, "Is there any way I can help?"

Four weeks ago, I sent a letter to my brother again. This time I wrote, "I'm going to tell you what I already told the rest of the family, I'm HIV positive and have been for the past eight years." I wrote him about how it affected me, how I had found a new meaning in life and was hoping that his need to punish me was less than his need to know his sister. I wrote him my phone number and added, "Call collect." He still hasn't been in touch.

This past Easter weekend, my mother invited me for the family lunch at the last minute. Usually, I'm not invited to my parents' for holidays because my brother doesn't want to run into me. This time, I was invited because he had cancelled. I felt like a fill-in. And I felt angry and rejected. I just refused the invitation, saying I was busy. After I put down the phone, I went out for a walk and had a cigarette. At that point, I hadn't smoked for two months. I was really disappointed with myself, but I know relapse is part of recovery.

Each relapse has been a lesson. This time, I felt betrayed because my mother wasn't saying, "Listen, Laura, I've invited Giles, but he cancelled and that gives me the perfect opportunity to see you." Then I would have gladly gone. Instead, she was so vague about it and just skirted around the issue. And I didn't have the courage to tell her how I felt.

Before, if I got into a tough place emotionally, I'd stop taking my pills. I don't do that now. I just relapsed with the smoking. Today, I eat well. I take my vitamins and my pills on time. And I'm going to stop smoking again. David jokes, "Don't stop smoking. You're a future customer." He sells respirators.

I met David seven years ago. A couple of nights a week, he and his friends met at the strip club after work for a beer. It was a neighbourhood club. We called them the SOB pack because they were all sons of bosses. The fathers were owners of the companies where they worked. I used to joke with David saying, "You're the only person I talk to who doesn't pay me." He showed me pictures of his children, one four years old and one eighteen months old. He talked to me about Judaism. I left Michael in October, and David applied for separation around the same time. A few months later we started seeing each other outside of the club.

After David and I came back from a weekend in Toronto, he thanked me for having gone away with him. I said, "Thanks for what? I didn't do anything."

He said, "Thank you for your spirit."

"My spirit?" That meant a lot to me. I know my light was out for a long time, and it seems like it's back.

I haven't told David about the HIV. I want to be with him, and I don't want to have this virus. I don't want to do this to him. How could I expect someone to wait around for what might be the inevitable? So I did what I did with Michael — told him I was going to be tested for

HIV and in three weeks, when I was supposed to get the results, I told him I tested positive.

When I told David I'm HIV positive, it was such a mess. But he had known for a year, long before we began to go out. He had heard about it from another stripper at the club, who had heard from Michael. Even though he had known, he freaked out when I told him. He was hoping against hope that it wasn't true. He said he didn't think I was the kind of person who would withhold such information. I said, "Well, you knew for a year, why didn't you just come out and ask me? I would have told you."

He said, "How do you ask a person a question like that?"

I said, "How do you tell a person something like that? We've been having such a good time that I didn't want it to end just because of the HIV."

After I told him, he went to get tested. During all this intrigue, the condom broke once. When I told him I was positive, he said, "That's it, I'm not sleeping with you till the results come back and even then, I don't know." Of course, his test came back negative.

That was a big lesson for me, the implications of what I did. It was all about manipulation. I was afraid to be honest.

I have no idea how to be a part of regular society, what I used to call the drones. What is normal and how normal do I want to be? What is it that a normal person wants? What are their goals, dreams and aspirations? And how do they attain them?

To understand normal has been very hard for me. To a church-going person, what I do is sinful. I don't feel it as a sin. I haven't done a fourth step on sexual misconduct because I believe that's between me and God, and it's not for man to pass judgement. I think lust makes me more aware of my fellow man. David is convinced I don't like my job. I said, "If it makes you feel better, I don't."

It would be unrealistic for me to go and apply for a job at an office because I have no experience in an office. But I do have plenty of experience in the sex trade. I'm usually one of the top three money-earners because I'm professional. Stripping is a nice income, and it's stable. I always have a job. Artistically, I'm probably one of the best strippers in the city. I usually get applause after every dance.

And not everyone does. I plan to continue till they no longer pay me.

I have a profession that offers me a great deal of freedom to express myself on stage. Not many people get to do cartwheels in the office. My image at work is that I'm a petite blond who's unpredictable. On stage, I put a tremendous amount of energy into my show, and I find transmitting the joy of life and living easy. When I talk to people one on one, I often talk about how good it feels to be alive. Yesterday I met someone who just got out of jail. I danced two songs for him and then gave him a big hug. I was able to caress his face, squeeze his knees, hold him, and tell him everything will be okay. It was very bittersweet.

I obviously can't do what I'm doing forever. I need to give myself some tools for later. The next part of my life will be devoted to people. I will be a teacher and a healer. Though I believe I have more healing work to do on myself before I can serve others.

There are changes I've made and insights I've had that are exclusive to me. I can be there for anyone with similar life experiences to mine in a way that no one else can. I'm the only person who can tell other junkies, other women with HIV, women who have been in battered situations, and alcoholics that it's okay, and know on a cellular level that it is.

I've been wanting to go back to school since I first got sober. Now, I'm enrolled at university in psychobiology. It's about how the psyche, environment, and food affects immunology. It's perfect for me. I'll get out of there with a B.Sc. I'll be able to work with people who have HIV and AIDS, teach them what I've learned about the spiritual aspect of life, and then give them a tangible: nutrition. Even if I end up getting sick, I'll be able to apply everything I'm learning to my own life. But through proper preventative measures, I won't have to succumb to this disease.

I'm going to get myself as educated as possible so that I can say, "Listen, this is how I extended my life so long." And the evidence of my being can be used to enhance someone else's life. I'm going to say this in proper scientific language so that I won't be discounted by physicians.

If you're going to live, there has to be something to live for. I need to have something to keep going for, and school is the perfect answer. I know the rest of the world sees me as dying, but people who are dying don't make plans for the future. It's important for me to make a contribution to society. I don't want to have lived here and not made a mark. It's the first time in my life that I've had a real direction that wasn't contingent on having hundreds of thousands of dollars, that wasn't a quick fix.

My New Year's resolution was to pace myself. I have to take an hour and a half each day to meditate. Meditation is very beneficial because the body is relaxed, and healing can only take place in a relaxed body. I have to provide three meals a day for myself. I go to three AA meetings a week. I immediately take care of any medical quirks. Before, I used to let things go. And I have to rest adequately. The longer I spend with myself and not feel lonely, the more I like myself. From here on, I'll always refine and grow, refine and grow.

Karen was never blessed with that insight and knowledge. She died of AIDS this Sunday. Besides talking to my mom about Easter, that was something else that happened on Sunday which made me return to smoking. Also, a week before Karen's death, a girl I had worked with at the club died of an overdose. That was a painful echo.

Karen and I were different, yet so alike. We were the same age. We were both junkies. We were both prostitutes. We were diagnosed with HIV around the same time. And I've been relatively comfortable, with only chronic yeast infections and low-grade fevers. She had it all.

Karen got HIV from a bisexual boyfriend who was into S&M and never told her he was infected. When she applied to nursing school, she was told to take an HIV test, which came back positive. She quit school and within a week was on the needle. I met her six years ago, when she had her first pneumonia. We became close because we had the same diagnosis and we used drugs together.

This past March, she said, "I'm not going to be here in April."

I said, "Karen, why are you giving up on yourself?"

She said, "I didn't give up on me, my doctor gave up on me."

I said, "Screw him, come to my doctor."

She said, "No, I'm just too tired."

That was when I let go of Karen because she had let go of herself. If she had been fighting till the very end, I would have been there for her. I would have fought with her. But she wrote herself off. And I just couldn't be there to watch it.

Seeing Karen in that box was a taste of reality for me. And it was twofold. First, that I have a killer disease, and second, that I am still walking. At her funeral, I realized that the reason I'm alive is because I had made some serious choices about my life.

I want to have lived before I die. I want to have a chance to really blossom. Karen never had a life. I don't want to die like that. I want to die knowing my work here is done. It's time to move on.

The beauty of having a terminal illness is that it gives you the chance to resolve everything. I don't have to carry any shit with me after I die. I will have had time to put all my affairs and relationships in order, and I'll be able to pass very peacefully at the time I decide to go. I do think death is a conscious decision. I'll know when it's the end, and I'll be ready.

I've had a recurring dream since I've been fifteen years old. In the dream, I know I'm one-hundred-and-four years old. I'm on the veranda of a house, sitting in a rocking chair and smoking a pipe. There are about twenty or thirty kids running in and out of the house. As a boy runs past me, I reach for the cane near my rocking chair and hit him on the ass with it, yelling, "Hey you, you need a haircut." The kid laughs and runs down the stairs. I collapse near the rocking chair and die.

I've had this dream about twenty or thirty times in my life, always the same dream, down to the detail of my wrinkled skin. So I always had the impression that I was going to die at the age of one hundred and four, surrounded by a lot of children.

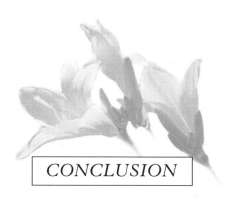

CONCLUSION

These portraits show that death, which most people view as negative, can also bring gifts. As I edited them, I was struck by certain threads and themes that emerged from apparently disparate lives.

Terminal illness has sharpened these people's awareness. Psychological problems have haunted them all their lives, and now these appear in relief. Florence confessed, "Fear has been my great vice." Bob admitted that he was "hiding everything." Laura said, "I was afraid to be honest." In hindsight, some people were able to see attitudes and attachments that they thought led to their illness. For Elaine, "The first cancer I believe was caused by the horrible last five years of my marriage. And the depression and sadness I had for that year and a half after Peter left caused the spread. . . . I had tremendous anger at the separation. I had invested in Peter." Both Sylvia and Elaine said they invested their hopes and dreams, as well as their labour, in the men they married; they had invested outside of themselves, in a mutable other, leaving themselves vulnerable.

As some of these people reflect on their lives, the theme of trying to be "perfect" crops up numerous times, specifically with Elaine, Sister Angela, Dianne, and Laura. Dianne observed, "I was never good enough, perfect enough." And later, "I had to learn to accept myself with all my imperfections. I now see that perfection isn't necessary.

Nor is it possible." Laura said, while talking about her past, "Anything other than perfection was not good enough."

When I asked if suffering can be viewed as positive, if it has a purpose, several people had asked themselves the same question. Florence's illness and her experience as a chaplain in an AIDS hospice had already raised this issue in her mind. She said, "I think that suffering is just a deepening that also has to do with character reformation. As we die, we have to work on the knots and kinks we've made in our character. It's a matter of purifying ourselves." Later she observed that "the deeper you suffer, the more you can enjoy, it's like mining space inside yourself to be able to hold more. Suffering cultivates an inner depth," and, "Suffering can take away the armour we have built to sustain our ego, to protect ourselves from others." Sister Angela said, "Suffering strengthens faith and trust." AIDS also made Dianne consider the question of suffering. She speculated, "I believe suffering can stretch people's limits. . . . [Through medical research] suffering has helped to better the human condition. It has been a catalyst to push us beyond our limits . . . both on a physical and psychological level, it has always helped people to evolve."

People seem to gain a greater appreciation of themselves and life as they feel death approaching. Claudine said, "I try to listen to myself. I'm learning that the most important person in this life is me. . . . Now my feelings are becoming more and more important." Later, she commented, "I have never before been as aware of people, myself, and life as I am now. . . . I have acquired a profound love of life because I've confronted death." Sylvia said, "I think for most of my life I didn't even allow myself to feel my own emotions. . . . now I have more time to pay attention." Sister Angela said, "When we say yes to death, we say yes to life ," and later, "I'm discovering that I can only really live when I can love myself." Laura declared, "I've had to become my own priority." Dianne said, "AIDS has allowed me to appreciate life as never before . . . and it's in this state of obvious imperfection that I have learned to finally appreciate myself. . . . Illness is a hard vehicle for growth, but sometimes that's what it takes." Bob said, "These past sixteen months have given me the opportunity to be with myself, to get to know myself. I've had time to think."

Surprisingly, some people did not want a cure for their disease. Bob said, "If they found a cure for AIDS tomorrow, I don't think I would take it." Claudine echoed these sentiments to the letter. They probably felt that what had been learned in this last phase of life might evaporate with a cure for their illness.

Facing death gave all of these people the courage to be honest and to pay attention to their needs. They all have a new sense of self; they all have had time to get to know and appreciate themselves. As Bob said, "The disease has allowed me to be myself. . . . Knowing that I am dying has given me a lot of courage. . . . I don't want to do things that I don't want to do anymore. . . . Before, I tolerated anything no matter how miserable I was." Sylvia observed, "This disease has taught me to value myself and has shown me that I'm a fighter. It's a paradox. I gain inner strength as my physical capacities diminish. . . . I have to live with the limitations of the illness, but I no longer have to live with the limitations others force upon me. . . . I'm more honest with myself and others." Sister Angela said, "This illness is giving me the time and opportunity to get to know myself better, in a way I have not yet done while serving Him. . . . Now I see that one of the most important feats in life is to accept oneself, to accept one's limits, one's needs, one's faults." Allan said, "This ridiculous situation has forced me to come face to face with myself."

They have all had to make changes in their lives since the illness, changes that most view in a positive light. Sylvia said, "I know the illness has actually served me. . . . The illness forced me to the edge."

Some become philosophical in this last phase of life. Keith said, "Man's nature is to ascend." Allan remarked, "For the first time in my life, I feel I'm taking an active role in my own evolution."

Awareness is important during all of life's stages, but particularly during the last one. Katherine enthusiastically observed, "It's important to pay attention when you feel your time has come and you're ready to die. . . . I don't want to miss anything."

Allan's response to the question, "Is it possible to have a sense of one's own death?" makes one stop and think: "If I can continue on the spiritual path I've begun, if I pay attention, I will know when the time approaches for me to die. And I will be prepared." Laura said,

"The beauty of having a terminal illness is that it gives you the chance to resolve everything. . . . I do think death is a conscious decision. I'll know when it's the end, and I'll be ready."

Finally, Dianne confirmed what I began to suspect when I had such a hard time finding dying people to interview: "If you have not healed your life . . . then dying must be very frightening." All these people have made profound efforts to do just that — heal their lives.

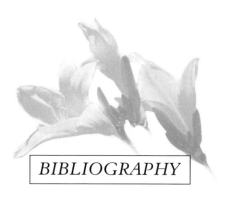

BIBLIOGRAPHY

Alexander, Franz, MD. *Psychosomatic Medicine*. New York: W.W. Norton, 1950.

Cameron, Jean. *Time to Live, Time to Die: A Health Care Professional Creatively Faces Her Own Terminal Cancer*. Hantsport, Nova Scotia: Lancelot, 1987.

Carroll, David. *Living With Dying: A Loving Guide for Family and Close Friends*. New York: McGraw Hill, 1985.

Chaney, Earlyne. *The Mystery of Death and Dying: Initiation at the Moment of Death*. York Beach, Maine: Samuel Weiser, 1988.

Choron, Jacques. *Death and Western Thought*. New York: Collier, 1963.

Cousins, Norman. *Head First: The Biology of Hope*. New York: Penguin, 1989.

Feuerbach, Ludwig. *Principles of the Philosophy of the Future*. Indianapolis: Bobs-Merrill, 1966.

Hay, Louise L. *The Aids Book: Creating a Positive Approach*. Santa Monica, California: Hay House, 1988.

Heidegger, Martin, tr. Joan Stambough. *Being and Time*. Albany: State University of New York, 1996

Jaspers, Karl, tr. J. Hoenig, Marian W. Hamilton. *General Psychopathology*. Manchester, England: Manchester University Press, 1963.

Jussek, Eugene G. *Reaching for the Oversoul*. York Beach, Maine: Nicolas-Hays, 1994.

Kalish, Richard A., ed. *Death, Dying, Transcending*. Farmingdale, New York: Baywood, 1980.

_____. *Death and Dying: Views from Many Cultures*. Farmingdale, New York: Baywood, 1980.

Kübler-Ross, Elisabeth. *On Death and Dying*. New York: Scribner Classics, 1997.

_____. *Life Lessons: Two Experts on Death and Dying Teach Us About the Mysteries of Life and Living*. New York: Scribner, 2000.

Levine, Stephen. *Meetings at the Edge: Dialogues with the Grieving and the Dying, the Healing and the Healed*. New York: Anchor, Doubleday, 1984.

_____. *Who Dies? An Investigation of Conscious Living and Conscious Dying*. New York: Anchor, Doubleday, 1982.

_____. *Healing into Life and Death*. New York: Anchor, Doubleday, 1987.

Morgan, Ernest. *Dealing Creatively with Death*. Bayside, New York: Zinn, 1994.

Northrup, Christine, MD. *Women's Bodies, Women's Wisdom: Creating Physical and Emotional Health and Healing*. New York: Bantam, 1998.

Saunders, Cicley M. *Living with Dying: The Management of Terminal Disease*. Oxford, England: Oxford University Press, 1983.

Shook, Robert L. *Survivors Living with Cancer: Portraits of Twelve Inspiring People*. New York: Harper and Row, 1983.

Shneidman, Edwin. *The Suicidal Mind*. New York: Oxford University Press, 1996.

_____. *Voices of Death: Letters and Diaries of People Facing Death — Comfort and Guidance for Us All*. New York: Kodansha American, 1995.

Simpson, Michael. *The Facts of Death*. Upper Suddle River, New Jersey: Prentice Hall, 1979.

Singer, June. *Seeing Through the Visible World: Jung, Gnosis and Chaos*. New York: Harper and Row, 1990.

_____. *Boundaries of the Soul: The Practice of Jung's Psychology*. New York: Anchor, 1994.

Sontag, Susan. *Illness as Metaphor*. New York: Farrar, Straus and Giroux, 1978.

Spark, Muriel. *Memento Mori*. London: Macmillan, 1959.

Steinem, Gloria. *Revolution from Within*. Boston: Little, Brown, 1992.

Walton, Douglas N. *On Defining Death: An Analytic Study of the Concept of Death in Philosophy and Medical Ethics*. Montreal: McGill-Queen's University Press, 1979.

_____. *Physician-Patient Decision Making: A Study in Medical Ethics*. Westport, Connecticut: Greenwood, 1985.

Viorst, Judith. *Necessary Losses*. New York: Simon and Schuster, 1998.

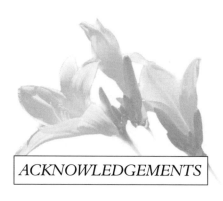

ACKNOWLEDGEMENTS

I would like to thank the Writers' Development Trust for their timely and generous help.

Infinite thanks to Isaak Hausmann, my father-in-law, who has supported the project in countless ways.

Gratitude to Dani, who had always backed my efforts and kept me in laughter through the crest and troughs this work entailed.

My appreciation to Ruth Bradley-St-Cyr, the godmother of this book. Thanks to Molly Fraser and Marie Thone for their help with the introduction and conclusion.

I would also like to express my debt to everyone who has helped along the way — spent time talking to me, allowing me to ponder aloud — nurses, doctors, social workers, and, the most valuable, the people who openly and generously answered my questions.